This Is Why You're
FAT

(And How to Get Thin Forever)

Old habits die hard. But what if your best (or what you *think* are your best) habits are to blame for the extra pounds you're packing? Spending hours on the treadmill, cutting fat intake, labeling certain foods "off-limits"—these are all behaviors that actually work *against* your body. Jackie's groundbreaking techniques for "tricking the brain" will change your body chemistry and the way you view your relationship with food forever. By simply changing your body chemistry with no-skimp nutrition and short workouts, plus thinking yourself thin, you will trim your body, tone your muscles, and get your best, hottest body ever! Now with her revolutionary plan, fitness guru Jackie Warner will show you how to work *with* your body to jump-start your motivation, kick your metabolism into high gear, and melt that fat away for good!

This Is Why You're
FAT

(And How to Get Thin Forever)

Eat More, Cheat More, Lose More— and Keep the Weight Off

JACKIE WARNER

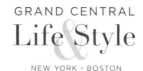

GRAND CENTRAL
Life & Style

NEW YORK • BOSTON

Copyright © 2010 by Jackie Warner

All rights reserved. In accordance with the U.S. Copyright Act of 1976, the scanning, uploading, and electronic sharing of any part of this book without the permission of the publisher is unlawful piracy and theft of the author's intellectual property. If you would like to use material from the book (other than for review purposes), prior written permission must be obtained by contacting the publisher at permissions@hbgusa.com. Thank you for your support of the author's rights.

Interior photos by Christopher Ameruoso

Grand Central Life & Style
Hachette Book Group
237 Park Avenue
New York, NY 10017

www.HachetteBookGroup.com

Grand Central Life & Style is an imprint of Grand Central Publishing.
The Grand Central Life & Style name and logo are trademarks of Hachette Book Group, Inc.

The Hachette Speakers Bureau provides a wide range of authors for speaking events. To find out more, go to www.hachettespeakersbureau.com or call (866) 376-6591.

The publisher is not responsible for websites (or their content) that are not owned by the publisher.

Printed in the United States of America

Originally published in hardcover by Grand Central Life & Style.

First Trade Edition: March 2012

10 9 8 7 6 5 4 3 2 1

The Library of Congress has cataloged the hardcover edition as follows:
Warner, Jackie, 1968–
    This is why you're fat (and how to get thin forever): eat more, cheat more, lose more—and keep the weight off / Jackie Warner.—1st ed.
        p.   cm.
ISBN 978-0-446-54860-1
1. Weight loss.   2. Reducing exercises.   I. Title.
RM222.2.W2784 2010

613.2'5-dc22   2009034641

ISBN 978-0-446-54858-8 (pbk.)

To my grandfather Jack Warner,
whom I was named after and to whom I attribute
the best in myself. I miss you every day.

Contents

Acknowledgments

Thanks to my literary agent, Mel Berger, and to my team at William Morris Agency for always looking out for my best interests and fighting the good fight. Thanks to Maggie Greenwood-Robinson for making sense out of my sometimes rambling thoughts. To Diana Baroni, my editor, who stayed positive and let me write the kind of book I wanted. Nicole Wool, you are an amazing publicist and so valued! Thanks to all of my friends at Bravo, specifically Cori Abraham, for always believing in me. Most of all, thanks to every individual who has reached out to me for guidance. You have made me a better teacher and a much better person.

THIS IS WHY YOU'RE FAT

(And How to Get Thin Forever)

Introduction

> ### *Being Fat Is a Problem, Staying Fat Is a Disaster*

This is a book for the fat and frustrated, for the sad and energy-challenged, and for all of you who know deep down that your life and body should be working better for you. I am not a doctor, dietitian, or psychologist; I *am* a fitness, nutrition, and energy specialist. I wrote this book because I have a deep desire to share my life's experiences and intense personal work to help you get thinner and happier. I'll do it by giving you knowledge and as many simple tools as possible to plug into your own life. Oh, and at forty, I have finally found the key to getting *my* hottest body, and higher levels of personal energy than ever before. So I can confidently say that yes, I have unlocked the secrets of how to get lean, healthy, and happy forever.

Let me just say this, too: I hate diet or fitness books that are complicated, elitist, and recommend stuff that's expensive or hard to find. Not everybody has access to top trainers, or amaranth grains, or special weight-loss herbs handed out by expensive Hollywood doctors. I wanted to write a book that breaks down the strongest, best-supported research principles into a program that *anyone* can follow, no matter what their shape, geographic location, or income level. In this book, you will find that program.

And it's a program that will give you what you really want: a hot and healthy body. I remember a client who weighed around three hundred pounds. Her heart, her blood sugar, her cholesterol—everything was a complete wreck. And she was addicted to prescription painkillers and antidepressants. As I gave her my speech that she would probably die from complications due to obesity, she looked me in the eye and said, "I don't care about all of that. I just want to walk into the Gap and buy a pair of jeans."

Okay. I get it. Scary statistics don't work in today's body-conscious culture. It's about you wanting to feel sexy in a bikini, tight jeans, or anything that comes in a smaller size. It's getting thin and healthy that matters. Some people are even saying: "Accept your fat." That's delusional. If you believe this, give it up. There's nothing loving, acceptable, or positive about eating your way to unattractiveness, fatigue, cancer, depression, and other terrible problems.

So yes, I get it, size is important to you. You care about your weight, and it's one of those numbers you keep tabs on. Clothing size, pounds on a scale, inches on a tape measure—all these numbers greatly impact your life. You feel great when you go down a size or two and horrible when you go up. It's that out-of-control roller-coaster ride that can affect your whole life. I'm going to show you how to get off that roller coaster and find stable ground.

I have a great advantage over most people because of the unique experience I gain through my work with thousands of clients at my gym. Such experience has led me to landing my national television show and forced me to stay on top of cutting-edge sports and nutrition science. But it was from my family background that I gained the most valuable advantage of all. I grew up in a dysfunctional family that struggled with depression, along with a number of chemical disabilities. My father was mentally ill with postwar schizophrenia and took his own life when I was eighteen. The challenges and pain from my childhood made me very empathetic to emotional struggles. I gained a strength that led me, through diet and exercise, to battle and cure my own depression, chronic fatigue syndrome, skin cancer, and, at times, crippling low-self-esteem issues.

As a kid, I was a sugar and junk-food addict. Comfort food was my drug of choice in dealing with emotional pain. I was thin, but was completely bingeing on mass quantities of processed food and sugar. And while no doctor told me, somewhere inside I knew it was causing my depression, learning disabilities, and terrible ADD. My teens and early twenties were filled with starvation diets followed by bouts of bingeing that left me feeling horrible about myself and out of control in my life—so much so that I even went to Overeaters Anonymous to combat my unhealthy relationship with food. Each diet I tried didn't work fast enough, or long enough, and led to feelings of failure and self-loathing.

Not until I reached my thirties and started really researching and applying the science of how the body changes with different foods, exercises, and metaphysical work did I finally turn the corner for good. I started adhering to a few commonsense rules for myself. These simple lifestyle changes have stuck with me and countless clients throughout the years.

Changing my lifestyle and my body has shown me that only *I* control my life and what it throws me. We all lose control and make bad decisions for ourselves. The key to weight loss and great self-esteem is decreasing the frequency of those mistakes. Losing control can be really fun in the moment, but almost always has negative long-term repercussions. This is true with anything in life, but especially with food. If you feel insecure and desperate about your body and eating habits, you are unhappy, and you must make a change in life *now* before your self-esteem is damaged so badly that it takes years to reverse. Trust me, it can be done. I've done it myself.

And you *will* do it with my eating and exercise program. It is so commonsense that you won't get confused, and your body will get so positively addicted to healthy food and exercise that you'll want to follow this program forever. It's different and better than anything out there.

Most of you reading this book have never been able to stick with a diet for more than a few months and never reached the goals you desired. Look, any great trainer can help you take off ten pounds of fat and push you to eat better. The problem is, the weight almost always comes back, and you fall into old patterns. My job is to give you all the information and secrets so that your weight stays off. Let me be very clear: You will learn how to achieve results and *stay* that way for as long as you *choose*. You will lose pounds and inches while gaining confidence and wellness. There are three simple rules in my program that will help you do that:

1. No overcomplicated diets or routines.

2. Deprivation does not work.

3. Live with intensity.

If you apply *any* three random principles from this book, your body will respond tremendously, and you will lose weight. These principles and disciplines have saved me, and pushed me to success and happiness.

On our life-changing journey together, you'll learn about the three forces that are making you fat: your body chemistry, sugar, and toxic organs. I will talk about all of these and tell you how you can overcome them. Being fat isn't your problem—meaning it's not totally your fault—but staying fat is! You can take control of these forces and take back your life and your weight. My program is like nothing you've ever done before. Here is what it offers.

Add Food to Lose Weight

Other diets take food out. Mine is the *only* diet that adds food in. These foods include natural, fat-burning foods that will help you get to your goals—and stay there. I will also tell you about all the body-killing, fat-storing foods to avoid. By adding certain foods in and subtracting offending foods, you won't ever crave any of the nasty stuff again. Expect your food cravings to almost disappear in two weeks!

Enjoy Hormone-Balancing Foods and Detox Foods

All the fad diets and "miracle" slimming products out there fail to recognize that weight gain is a result of out-of-whack hormones, excess sugar, and poorly functioning organs. When you address these things, you will succeed. My program shows you how to balance your hormones through diet and exercise, ease off sugar, and detox the organs responsible for fat loss. This approach makes weight loss easy, because you're giving your body what it really craves—balance. On my program, you'll eat better, feel better, look better, and become happier. Your body will become a fat-burning machine!

Be a Weekend Cheater

Here's one of the best parts of my program: You eat clean (healthy foods) for five days and enjoy two treat meals on the weekend. Yes, you get to "cheat" for *two* meals! My clients love this about my program. Sure, some programs allow one treat meal a week. I know human nature, and one treat meal a week is not gonna cut it for the rest of your life. So during the week, you'll eat like you're at work, knowing the light's at the end of the tunnel on the weekend!

My program is not about punishing yourself. It's about giving yourself permission to have less-than-healthy foods for two meals, with the understanding that you'll spend the rest of the week eating hormone-balancing and detox foods to burn fat. This is how I eat and live. On the weekends, I allow myself ice cream, a martini, or candy at the movies. This is so doable, you'll be surprised at how easy it is. And guess what? After five days of clean eating, your brain doesn't have the same desire for junk food! This is one of the secrets to long-term weight loss: tricking the brain not to feel deprived. With my program, you will naturally stop wanting the large quantities of food you used to eat . . . without any thought!

Eat More

Give up starvation diets. They ruin your metabolism. Many of the heaviest people who come to me have one thing in common: They try to starve themselves down to size by skipping meals. That will get you nowhere fast, except into a larger size and a permanently slow metabolism. *Deprivation does not work!* Nutrient deprivation is responsible for much of your weight gain. When you skip meals, your body thinks it's being starved, so it slows your metabolism and stores fat it would normally burn. And the next time you eat, your body will store fat almost twice as fast. On my program, you eat more than before, not less, and that means five times a day. Eating hormone-balancing and detox foods throughout the day is a key to getting thin.

Look and Feel Great

You want to be thin—and gorgeous. Well, the two go hand in hand. The things that will help you drop sizes are the same things that will make you look beautiful. See, to make the most of your hair, skin, and nails, you've got to give up the trans fats, cheap sugars, excess sodium, and unpronounceable additives dumped into junk food. This stuff is ugly—and it makes you ugly, fat, and wrinkled.

You've got to feed your body the best possible stuff—like protein (lean meats), fruits and veggies, and whole grains (like brown rice). Skip them and you'll never even know your beauty potential. The foods on my program will give you flawless skin, a toned body, and tons of energy. They will also de-age you. I guarantee that if you follow my program, people will tell you that you look younger and more attractive.

Get Thin in the Real World

I used to tell overweight clients exactly what to eat and when to eat and exercise. They would do great for a couple of months, then fall off the wagon, wanting to throw in the towel. I couldn't figure out why, so I started asking a lot of questions. It came down to this: I had to take all the thinking out of dieting and exercising. I had to be more realistic about what life is like in their world. I couldn't force-feed my organic, highly disciplined way of eating to everyone. Real life consists of restaurants, after-work drinks, junk food in the house for the kids, job and financial pressures, skinny spouses who eat whatever they want, oh, and depression from not being fulfilled. On my program, you will learn how to choose the good—veggies, fruit, and lean proteins; avoid the bad—starches and bread; and skip the ugly—desserts and alcohol. All this at the grocery store and at restaurants.

Burn with Intensity

My exercise program is designed to speed up your metabolism and add lean muscle *super-fast*—without spending hours in the gym. Workout sessions don't need to be long; they should be strong and intense. My own brand of intense exercise combinations will give you maximum benefit and results. They burn fat faster and add muscle to speed up your metabolism. You'll never, ever get bored with this workout, because each time you challenge yourself to perfect your form and increase your weights. There *are* ways to maintain the passion in your fitness program, and I'll give them to you. All of my training secrets are here, including what will truly give you sexy abs. And by the way, crunches are a waste of time, and I'll tell you why.

Have More Energy

We are a nation of sick, unhealthy people wasting away and mutating into sad, fat, and lethargic people, just getting fatter and sadder by the second. We are an out-of-control nation with out-of-control waistlines. I have noticed that a mass panic is setting in. I see it every day in the faces of people and desperate e-mails from around the country. So many people are tired, always dragging and feeling exhausted. Many are a walking medicine chest, dependent on pills to control everything from high blood pressure to sleep deprivation, and are chronically fatigued and depressed. Others can't climb a flight of stairs or walk a block without gasping for air. Millions of people are alive, but hardly living.

I realize you care mostly about getting thin, not about cholesterol levels. But who wants to be sick, tired, and depressed when you don't have to be? Bagfuls of doughnuts or chips are not worth lessening the quality of your life or shortening it.

The effects of poor nutrition and a lack of exercise not only are visible on the outside but will wipe you out on the inside. It's time to take responsibility and treat your body as the greatest gift you have. It is your calling card to life, and through its energy, you can shine as the person you were always meant to be. The foods you'll learn to eat here and the exercise you'll do will help transform your life in every way.

Take Back Your Self-Control

I believe that self-control is what we all long for, yet it is something that can come only from within. What interferes with self-control is constant worry and obsession over food and weight. You should not worry about food and your weight all day long! This is not normal. It's exhausting, and it takes energy away from more creative, positive thoughts about yourself and your environment. Eating should energize you—not stress you out—and free you! On every page of this book, I cut through all the confusion and talk about *freedom*. Freedom from constantly thinking of food, freedom from negative body image, and freedom from all the drama attached to not being happy with your circumstances.

When you're struggling with your weight, you also carry a load of negative feelings: disappointment, frustration, self-loathing, and not measuring up. To make things worse, these feelings make you want to eat because you equate food with comfort. Food becomes a way to self-medicate from an unhappy life. Not to mention that it's impossible to do everyday things without being bombarded by junk food and struggling with whether to eat it or not eat it. These constant internal battles kill self-control and positive self-esteem.

The solution is nutrition and exercise! You won't start feeling comfortable and connected with yourself until you have control over both. Then you'll gain control over your body and your life. When you put clean, energy-giving foods into your system, and exercise with intensity, your body produces positive body chemicals. These chemicals change how you look and feel. They allow you to radiate high energy that attracts into your world anything you want—the ability to get thin, build self-esteem, achieve success—anything.

Think Fit, Be Fit

What goes on in your head is usually 100 percent responsible for weight gain! I'm going to show you how to throw out the junk in your head, because how you think defines who you are. We all have deeply rooted traits that drive us to succeed or fail in life. Enough small and consistent success leads to inner peace and happiness. Too many failures left unchecked may lead to self-loathing and an unsatisfied life.

In this book, I will show you that it's never too late to reinvent yourself and work against "bad" genetics, or your created environment. So to make a change, you must begin thinking differently. Decide that your appearance, health, and fitness are as important as anything else. Your body naturally wants to be thin. You have the power to make that happen. I will share key secrets with you that will give you simple tools to reframe your thinking and still achieve your biggest goals while dealing with life's setbacks. Whether you're a mom juggling a thousand things, or a busy professional with deadlines and other added stressors, every day is an opportunity to feel amazing about yourself!

Feel Powerful in Your World

In life we all need friends, motivators, and teachers to boost us up and inspire us when we are unable to inspire ourselves. That's what I can be for you. My job is to empower you to make a lasting, lifelong change. Your job is to redefine what working out, relationships with food, and overall happiness in your life will be.

As a trainer, I push people ten times harder than they ever thought they could go. They give it to me, and afterward, they feel like a million bucks. That's what I'm passionate about: showing people how powerful they really are. I've discovered that we trainers may be more like therapists than any other profession. When you deal with the body, there's a lot of pain people keep inside, and a lot is based on how they feel about themselves from an early age. I have to be empathetic and a good listener, as well as knowing what I'm talking about. I've changed clients' lives—gotten them into AA and out of marriages, seen them through babies and deaths and new careers. These changes start, however, when they lose weight and keep fit. The *product* of what I do is a good-looking body, but the *by-product* is more energy, job satisfaction, better sex—everything in life gets better. That's what it's all about for me. I'm not interested in helping some celebrity get an eight-pack. I want to help people better their lives.

You *deserve* to be lean, strong, happy, and confident in the way you look, the way you feel, and the way you live. I want for all of you to experience waking up every morning feeling sexy, strong, and powerful in your body. There's nothing like it, trust me. It is time *you* start feeling powerful in *your* world.

And it's time to take small, yet significant steps in the right direction, and set yourself on a better path. Your lifestyle is determined by what you put in and do with your body . . . period. I promise that I will give you the right information, in the right way, to help you make the right choices for yourself and see enormous differences in your life. We make a choice every day to get either strong or weak. Let this be your day to get strong. The best decision that you can make right now is to be the best you can be.

It's also time to ignite a fire within that leads to not only a hot body, but also great self-worth and confidence. Know that it's impossible to live perfect in an imperfect world, so stop beating yourself up! Just start to make one positive choice each day, and you will find your days getting better.

And if you've identified yourself as "the fat girl or guy" your entire life, but are ready to get thin, you are my hero. The bravery it takes to walk into a gym, trust, do the work, and redirect your thinking is something I admire tremendously. I see achievers like you every day in my gym. Their struggle touches me deeply and is very relatable to everyone who has had to fight against society, their families, and the worst critic—themselves. I love being a part of their journey—and yours.

Your body is a science project, and you can change it in twenty-four hours. Know that right now, in this one, single day, your body has already started its change for the better, because your focus there has allowed it to. All you need is this book, a measuring tape, and your journal, and you can take your life back.

Nothing you do or try is ever a failure, just an opportunity to make a bigger change and grow. Every day is a new starting point. Keep your eye on the prize: a leaner, happier, healthier you!

Let's go!

Part 1

THIS IS WHY YOU'RE FAT

1 It's All About Chemistry, Baby

Let's start talking about why you're fat. Fat control has largely to do with hormones. I always knew that hormones played a large part in how we feel, but I never dreamed that they were so responsible for metabolizing fat and maintaining muscle. Take testosterone, for example. The hormone testosterone is the reason, ladies, that your husbands and boyfriends can eat whatever they want and not gain a pound, while you count calories and can't lose a pound.

My extreme interest in hormones happened in my late thirties after I went to my doctor, complaining that I felt tired and didn't have the energy for my usual exercise routine. He did my blood work and found that I was terribly low in progesterone. My blood sugar was also low. I learned that low blood sugar is a precursor to diabetes, which runs in my family, and I learned that low progesterone causes sleeplessness and fatigue.

None of this was acceptable to me, so I started to research natural ways to balance my blood sugar and my hormones. As I researched, I was astonished to find out how much cutting-edge data linked weight management to hormones! Out-of-whack hormones

> ## In This Chapter:
>
> * Three hormones that make you thin
> * Four hormones that make you fat
> * Balance your hormones naturally
> * Outsmart cravings
> * Get rid of cellulite

disturb your body chemistry and cause weight gain. When you control your hormones, you can control fat!

Hormones, of course, are powerful chemicals and a crucial part of your inner environment. They impact every area of your life—how you feel, how you act and react, and how you look. When hormones are nicely balanced, your health is great. You enjoy strength, energy, and beauty. But when hormones shift and fluctuate, things can get pretty ugly. Having hormone dysfunction feels like you are constantly fighting a battle and never winning the war. You have constant cravings for unhealthy food, you feel slightly lethargic and depressed, and you don't have the energy for a real workout.

There are actually four hormones responsible for making you fat and three hormones responsible for making you thin. The secret is to have all seven in balance and operating as they should. That's when you'll truly lose weight, without a lot of painful sacrifices, and keep it off. I'm going to tell you what all these hormones are, how they work, and how lifestyle affects their balance, so that you can get thin and healthy. Here's the deal.

Hormones That Make You Thin

Human Growth Hormone: The Fountain of Youth

One of the greatest get-thin hormones is human growth hormone (HGH). It's a fat burner that works in the following manner: Normally, your body uses glucose (blood sugar) for energy before it taps into fat for energy. But HGH reprioritizes everything. It forces your body to draw energy from your fat reserves first. This turns you into a fat-burning machine, even during inactive periods like when you're sleeping. With plenty of HGH in your system, you don't have to diet all the time.

Another great benefit of HGH is that it helps your body to grow new muscle cells. Normally, you stop making muscle cells after your teen years. If you do resistance training, you'll increase the size of the muscle cells you do have. The number of muscle cells never grows, however, unless there's adequate HGH in your body. So HGH helps you get toned and sculpted by creating more muscle cells.

HGH also gives you more energy, a higher sex drive, and youthful skin and hair. HGH is truly a wonder hormone.

But here's the challenge: HGH starts plummeting through our thirties and forties, making it harder to get toned and look lean. Luckily, diet and exercise actually boost HGH levels, allowing it to rejuvenate and beautify your body.

So how can you naturally raise your hormone levels? It's not as hard as it may seem. Here's how I did it.

CUT BACK ON CARBS AT NIGHT

When blood sugar is low, your body pumps out more HGH. The best way to capitalize on this situation is to keep your carbohydrate intake low in the evening. For dinner, have protein and some low-carb veggies, but no carbs like bread, pasta, rice, or potatoes. HGH will then accelerate fat loss by mildly increasing your metabolism and boosting muscle growth while you sleep.

GET A GOOD NIGHT'S SLEEP

And while I'm talking about sleep, you should know that sleep deprivation almost completely abolishes HGH production. Deep sleep is when the body produces HGH—so you've got to get a good night's sleep every night. What I've found is that eating casein-rich foods like low-fat cottage cheese will help you sleep. Also, don't drink caffeine products past three o'clock, and never sleep with your television on.

EAT HGH BUILDING BLOCKS

These include foods high in the B vitamins, like whole grains, legumes, vegetables, and proteins; the mineral zinc, found in lean proteins; and any protein-rich food. My nutrition program is packed with these nutrients, so you will automatically be eating HGH building blocks.

GO ORGANIC

Many of our foods are loaded with pesticides and chemicals, which lower HGH. To avoid these body-killing substances, eat as many organic foods as you can. I'll have more to say on this in chapter 6.

TRAIN HARD

Intense workouts improve your body chemistry, including levels of HGH. Sprinting and weight training, both of which are intense training modes, have been shown to increase HGH release, improving your metabolism. The intensity of the training you'll do on my program will help trigger greater HGH release.

But what about those over-the-counter supplements and pills promising to boost the production of growth hormone sold in health-food stores and over the Internet? There's no evidence that pills work. Rejuvenation centers sell injectable HGH, but it is very costly and may have some dangerous side effects. So forget pills and injections. Rely on natural ways to increase HGH.

Testosterone: The Muscle Builder

My favorite hormone is testosterone, made in the ovaries and adrenal glands. While mostly associated with men, testosterone is critically important for women. It builds muscle, burns fat, boosts energy, increases sex drive, strengthens bone, lifts depression, and increases optimistic thinking. In women who have normal to high testosterone levels, it produces assertiveness—which is why I know my body produces it in spades.

The aging process makes testosterone levels drop. So do lifestyle factors like diet, alcohol use, smoking, stress levels, and your overall state of health. But this doesn't mean you're helpless. You can make your body produce more testosterone in the following ways.

EAT TESTOSTERONE BUILDERS

These include foods rich in beta-carotene (yellow and orange vegetables and green leafy veggies); foods high in B vitamins (found in a wide range of foods like beef, green leafy vegetables, and other veggies); and foods containing boron (fruits, nuts, and legumes). All of these foods cause your body to produce more testosterone. Other testosterone boosters are amino acids. Amino acids are the building blocks of cells, antibodies, muscle tissue, and enzymes. They're found mostly in protein foods such as eggs, poultry, fish, and meats, as well as in certain dietary supplements.

WATCH FAT INTAKE

A typical high-fat American diet alters testosterone levels. The journal *Modern Medicine* conducted a study looking into this. Eleven healthy men, ages twenty-three to thirty-five, who ate a daily, high-fat eight-hundred-calorie meal of a shake containing 57 percent fat, experienced a dramatic 30 percent drop in testosterone levels. Could the same effect occur in women? Medical researchers believe so, since testosterone production relies on the right balance of fat in the diet—not too high, not too low.

If you really want testosterone to make you thin, you do need some fat in your diet, even a little bit of saturated (animal) fat. Saturated fats are essential for keeping testosterone levels up, but they also get stored preferentially as body fat. To get around this and still obtain the testosterone-building benefits, limit your red meat intake to three servings per week and eat more poultry and fish. Eating more monosaturated fats (from nuts, olive oil, avocados) and polyunsaturated fats (fatty fish) is a good idea, too, because they're burned for fuel, and they don't make you fat (unless of course you overdose on them). The best testosterone diet is a healthy moderate-fat/high-protein/moderate-carb diet—which is how my nutrition program works. This type of diet creates a hormonal environment in the body that burns fat and puts on lean muscle.

WATCH CAFFEINE AND ALCOHOL

How much caffeine and alcohol you consume affects your testosterone levels. Drinking more than two cups of coffee or four cans of caffeinated soda a day will make your testosterone levels drop. Ease back on alcohol, too. Frequent drinking blunts testosterone production.

Progesterone: The Slim and Trim Hormone

The third fat-burning hormone you want to balance is progesterone. High levels of progesterone burn more calories—as much as one hundred to three hundred per day! Progesterone is a natural diuretic that reduces bloating. It also helps prevent uterine fibroids and cancer, improves libido, and boosts mental clarity.

Every month, after an egg is released, your body secretes progesterone. If you don't get pregnant, progesterone levels plunge, triggering a slow metabolism and low blood sugar. When your blood sugar dips, you crave food—usually high-sugar or sweet food—so it's no wonder you can't lose weight! Low progesterone also causes insomnia, disrupted sleep, and daytime sleepiness. Now is the time to change your diet and include lots of progesterone-enhancing foods that will make you sleep better and metabolize fat. Balancing progesterone is key to avoiding weight gain and energy drains.

INCLUDE PROGESTERONE-BUILDING FOODS

For optimal progesterone production, your body needs lots of B vitamins, in particular vitamin B_6. It's found in beans, meat, poultry, fish, and some fruits and vegetables, like bananas, avocados, spinach, and tomatoes. The other key nutrient in progesterone production is magnesium. Eat plenty of organic dark green leafy vegetables, almonds, eggs, meat, seeds, nuts, and beans. They are all good sources of magnesium, and they also keep your liver healthy. Poor liver function suppresses progesterone. Once you get started on my program, you'll find that it works in harmony with the body's metabolism and ability to make hormones, including progesterone, that regenerate the body.

Four Hormones That Make You Fat

Insulin: Spikes Make You Fat

Insulin is the hormone that, under normal conditions, turns food into energy. But if there's too much insulin in your system, your body will store fat, and much of what you eat gets packed away as ugly pounds. And the bigger you get, the more insulin your body cranks out. It's a vicious cycle. How does insulin get too high, anyway, and what can you do to keep it in line?

Insulin rises and falls according to what you eat, particularly carbs. All carbs, whether they're from chocolate or whole-grain bread, break down in the body into glucose, or blood sugar, which is the fuel for your muscles and brain. Sugary carbs like cookies and some processed starches (such as pasta and white bread) are broken down into glucose rapidly; proteins and fats break down more gradually.

The arrival of glucose in the bloodstream signals the pancreas to make insulin. Sugary foods dump so much glucose into the blood so fast that the pancreas has to pump out extra insulin to drive glucose into cells. Blood sugar levels dip lower than they were before the sugar was eaten. This leads to hunger pangs and eating when we don't actually need to. Once a hunger pang hits, it's too late! Your insulin has already dropped so low that the next thing you put in your mouth will be effectively stored away as fat. Insulin spikes and dips make you fat.

Judith Rodin, a pioneering researcher in the psychological and physiological factors of obesity, did an experiment in which she had people drink sugar water to purposely spike their insulin levels. With high insulin, the volunteers actually ate five hundred calories more in one meal! Some studies show that even the sight of sugary, fatty foods can cause an insulin spike that starts a craving in your mind. So the saying "Just looking at those cupcakes makes me fat" is true!

If you eat processed and high-sugar foods (this means breads, too) long enough, your body can become less sensitive to insulin and require more of it just to get glucose escorted into cells. This situation is called insulin resistance. If you're insulin-resistant, your body isn't moving the food you eat into your muscles. About 25 percent of all adults are insulin-resistant. One in two people have it if they're older than forty-five—and overweight.

Insulin resistance is nasty. It causes fatigue, mood swings, memory loss, and weight gain. It makes you sick, with terrible diseases like type 2 diabetes, high blood pressure, Alzheimer's disease, stroke, heart disease, and cancer.

Fortunately, you can eat your way out of insulin problems. If you add in just one right food like oatmeal, in place of one bad food like a bagel, your insulin levels will start to fall right way. There are other foods that, if eaten on the right schedule, will produce an even flow of glucose that will keep you satisfied. You won't need superhuman willpower to lose fat, because your body won't feel any cravings. Exercise drives insulin levels down, too. Once you start following my program, your insulin levels will normalize, and your body will stop storing fat.

CRAVINGS: THE CHEMISTRY BEHIND SELF-DESTRUCTIVE EATING

WHETHER YOU'RE REALLY HEAVY or ten to twenty pounds overweight, you know what a struggle it is to try to control your cravings. You may succeed for a few days, but then you just can't stop yourself. This is not a matter of willpower. It's a chemistry problem.

Cravings are a sudden obsession with a particular type of food—and they're triggered mostly by messed-up body chemistry. When levels of the hormone estrogen fall, for example, levels of the brain neurotransmitter serotonin drop, and appetite increases. And when insulin is too high, you'd kill for a cookie, or maybe a whole box. This is why it's so hard to just eat a little bit of something sweet. Your brain is signaling your body to crave more and more of the snack.

Dr. Judith J. Wurtman, a nutritionist at MIT, has shown that eating refined carbs like cake, candy, cookies, or white bread raises serotonin and endorphins in the brain, creating a happy, peaceful state—which is why you turn to carbs when you're anxious and stressed. These spikes of happy hormones make you calm only in the short term, however. You are literally self-medicating with food.

Some people crave sweets and others, bread. It doesn't matter, because it all converts quickly to sugar in your body and feeds the cravings more. Fortunately, you can trick your system not to be hungry. Some tips to satisfy cravings the smart way:

* Reach for fruit when a craving hits. Fruit is your best defense against insulin spikes and the resulting cravings.

* Be prepared. If you know that the afternoon is when you're likely to crave junk, stash healthy snacks in your desk, like carrots, nuts, a low-cal protein bar, celery with peanut butter, hard-boiled eggs, or prepackaged foods under 150 calories and five grams of sugar.

* Beware of high-protein diets like Atkins. These ultimately fail because they cause serotonin levels in the brain to fall sharply. You'll feel moody as a result, and want to reach for sweets and refined carbs as an antidote.

* Move your body. People who exercise regularly rarely have cravings. Why? Working out helps rebalance your hormones and increases feel-good chemicals in your body.

Estrogen: Balance This Hormone and Be Thin

Estrogen is a wonderful hormone. In the right amount, it makes conception and pregnancy possible. It's also a natural mood lifter and skin toner.

Estrogen works in sync with progesterone, and both hormones need to be in balance. Progesterone is the estrogen police; it helps balance estrogen. In the right ratio, the two hormones help the body burn fat for energy, act as an antidepressant, assist metabolism, and promote sleep. When your body doesn't have enough progesterone to keep the estrogen in check, you become estrogen-dominant. Unfortunately, in America, we become estrogen-dominant in another way: We are fed foods that cause the problem.

Estrogen dominance can wreak havoc. Too much estrogen in our bodies leads to weight gain, cellulite, and some female cancers. It also slows down your thyroid gland (which controls metabolism). Your metabolic rate drops like mad. There's more: Estrogen causes water and salt to be retained in bodily tissues. This makes you look soft and spongy. This type of serious bloat not only makes you look bad, but also activates an enzyme that makes your body store fat. You can gain ten to fifty pounds of fat! A young woman can have the slow, screwed-up metabolism of a menopausal woman. Estrogen dominance can also cause anxiety, brain fog, low sex drive, and poor blood sugar control.

Environmental toxins, rampant stress, nutritional deficiencies, and the estrogens leaching into our food supply have turned America into an estrogen-dominant society. Here are a few things that can cause estrogen dominance:

* Processed foods or foods rich in sugar (this includes bread products such as crackers or bagels, too). Processed foods are practically devoid of fiber, and you need fiber in your diet. Fiber from natural foods like whole grains, fruits, and vegetables moves estrogen out of the body. Without enough dietary fiber, estrogen builds up and increases the hormonal burden on your system.

* Alcohol and caffeine. Having more than two cups of coffee per day increases estrogen. Alcohol impedes the liver's ability to metabolize estrogen. When the liver fails to break down estrogen, it stays in the body and makes you fat.

* Estrogen compounds are fed to chickens and cattle to increase meat, egg, and dairy production. These estrogens can then get passed on to us when we eat meat, eggs, and poultry, or drink milk. Our bodies are becoming a stew of excessive estrogen stimulation, and it's wrecking our health!

* Some plastics. Heating up plastics, either by microwaving foods in plastic containers or drinking hot beverages out of plastic cups, releases bisphenol A (BPA), an estrogen compound. BPA then leaches into the food, causing estrogen to be produced. So think twice before heating plastic containers in the microwave or drinking out of plastic cups. When buying bottled water, look for containers that have a number 7 in their recycling code; those don't usually contain BPA.

Under normal conditions, hormones do their jobs properly. They're disassembled by the body and removed from the bloodstream. Environmental estrogens that we ingest from the food supply or get from plastics, however, tend to stay in the body and remain active for much longer periods, where they promote estrogen dominance and make you gain weight. To stabilize your body's levels of estrogen, you need to reduce its production and assist its breakdown and elimination—all of which you can do by undertaking a natural approach. Here are some suggestions.

EAT HORMONE-FRIENDLY

Eliminate sugar and highly processed foods. Look for organic meat and dairy products that are certified free of hormones. Boost

---

ARE YOU ESTROGEN-DOMINANT?

IF THREE OR MORE of these statements fit you, you may be estrogen-dominant and should have your hormone levels tested.

I'm older than thirty-five.

I've been gaining weight for no apparent reason.

I have noticeable cellulite.

I suffer from premenstrual syndrome (PMS).

My periods are heavy and irregular.

I am often anxious, irritable, and moody.

My eyes and face are often puffy.

I've been losing interest in sex.

I have trouble sleeping.

My body retains water.

I have frequent headaches.

I often feel forgetful.

My breasts sometimes feel lumpy.

My breasts sometimes feel tender.

your intake of whole grains, plant-based proteins, good fats, colorful fruits and vegetables, green tea, and good sweeteners like Truvia, which is a stevia-based sweetener. Stevia is an herb that has been commercialized as a natural sweetener. It is approximately three hundred times sweeter than sugar and has a negligible effect on blood sugar levels.

Drink with Care

Water (three liters daily) helps cleanse your liver and kidneys, allowing your body to excrete hormones efficiently. Avoid caffeinated beverages; while caffeine produces an initial lift, it also stimulates the adrenal glands to produce more cortisol (a stress hormone), worsening anxiety, fatigue, and other symptoms. As for alcohol, consuming too much can compromise the liver's ability to metabolize estrogen, which can cause estrogen levels to rise. Minimize its use or avoid it altogether.

Keep Stress in Check

When women are under severe stress, they're less likely to ovulate. If you don't ovulate, you don't produce progesterone during the second half of your cycle. Without enough progesterone to keep estrogen in check, the negative effects of estrogen can become more pronounced. Stress also raises levels of cortisol, which causes other hormones to get out of balance, and decreases testosterone. Starting a positive and life-changing new program can relieve stress and give you an attitude shift. Stress relief starts when you take control over your life!

Cortisol Creates Stress Fat

Speaking of stress, if you stay stressed out, you're working against your body's natural desire to stay thin and healthy! Cortisol is made in the adrenal glands and is the hormone that helps regulate blood sugar, the movement of carbohydrates, proteins, and fats into and out of the cells, and muscle function.

A single bout of stress—say, you swerve to avoid a collision on the highway—causes your cortisol level to surge instantly, but it soon returns to normal. Cortisol is meant to help your body respond appropriately to these occasional short-lived alarms. Chronic stress, however, is an unnatural state for the body, and when it's sustained or frequently repeated, cortisol levels get jammed in high gear.

When exposed to chronic stress, the body is bathed in a flood of cortisol, leading to higher insulin levels and an around-the-clock appetite, typically for sweets and fatty foods. Elevated cortisol stockpiles calories, storing them in fat cells in the tummy for future use. It also causes a drop in the brain chemical serotonin, leading to depression, irritability, and cravings.

Elevated cortisol levels can cause thinning skin, muscle wasting, memory loss, high blood pressure, dizziness, hot flashes, excessive facial hair, and other masculinizing tendencies. That's not so hot, is it? I know it's so hard to live stress-free, but you can change *what* you stress over. You may not be able to control what happens at work or who does what to you, but you do have control over how you respond. Take an active role in balancing your body, and stop freaking out about your weight and food all the time. A healthy response to stress will make you naturally feel less stressed out. A fit and healthy person can easily deal with spiked cortisol, but an unhealthy dieter will gain a slow metabolism.

The good news is you can keep all cortisol hell from breaking loose by eating regular, healthy meals. Foods that keep cortisol in check include casein-rich cottage cheese, green leafy vegetables, whole-grain breads, mushrooms, and fruits, especially berries. Exercise keeps cortisol from taking over your body.

Self-medicating with alcohol, tobacco, caffeine, sugar, and over-the-counter drugs to control stress is just masking your stress instead of managing it. Stop the use of these "pick-me-ups" and you'll get a consistent feeling of well-being. One month into my program and you'll be less dependent on these things. I have seen it time and again with all of my clients. Your body will naturally start rejecting the bad things you used to rely on. With better habits in place, you'll be less thrown by cortisol—and you'll start naturally losing weight.

Leptin: Tame Your Appetite

The fat cells in your body produce a hormone called leptin. At adequate levels, leptin works as an appetite suppressant. In other words, it tells your brain when it's time to stop shoving fries in your face. It also keeps your metabolism high and averts drops in testosterone.

But when levels are too low, leptin signals your body to store fat. So obviously, you want to keep levels of leptin high in your body, and there are ways to do that naturally.

EASE BACK ON ASIAN FOOD

Yes, it's often greasy, but that's not the only reason it can pack on pounds. According to a study in *Obesity,* people who eat lots of monosodium glutamate (MSG) are twice as likely to be overweight as those who rarely eat foods with the flavor enhancer. This is because MSG may lower levels of leptin. Next time you order at an Asian restaurant, have them hold the MSG. And check ingredients in foods: MSG is often listed as "hydrolyzed protein."

LOG ENOUGH ZZZS

Your body produces leptin while you sleep, so skimping on sleep can drastically lower levels.

EAT SLOWLY

It takes approximately twenty minutes for leptin to kick in, and you start feeling full. Eat part of your meal, stop, drink a glass of water, wait a few minutes, then continue eating the rest. This trick is especially helpful over the holidays or at restaurants, when there's more food around to tempt you.

EAT FISH

Seafood is known to raise leptin levels in the body, because of the omega-3 fatty acids it contains. Shoot for at least two to three fish meals a week. Not everyone likes fish, of course. An alternative is to supplement with omega-3s. Take one to three grams a day with food.

GET IN SYNC WITH ZINC

Being deficient in zinc results in less leptin. Women need at least nine milligrams daily of this energy-boosting mineral, the amount in most multi-vitamin-mineral tablets. Zinc-rich foods include poultry and seafood.

> ### FAT-BURNING FACT: LEPTIN HIBERNATES IN WINTER
>
> **DOES YOUR APPETITE** get ravenous when the temperature plunges? Blame it on leptin. According to a recent study, some people may not process leptin as efficiently during the winter, causing them to gain weight. Experts aren't sure why this is the case, but they agree that better leptin production can curb your appetite and make you feel fuller.
>
> *Source: The National Institute of Mental Health*

* * *

The bottom line is that out-of-whack hormones make you fat and keep you fat. Manipulate your hormones and improve your body chemistry through the right foods and exercise, and expect to lose pounds. Once you begin my program, you'll discover how easy it is to get your hormones under control and manage your weight. You're the boss of your hormones.

CELLULITE SUCKS!

WOULDN'T IT BE NICE to have a dimple-free butt and thighs? But as we age, our bodies tend to develop cellulite. Cellulite is fat that gets trapped between fibers that connect your muscles to your skin. The fibers are like the stitching on a down quilt— cellulite puffs out between them. The more fat you have between fibers, the more visible your cellulite tends to be.

Blame cellulite mostly on estrogen. It causes fat storage in the hips, thighs, and butt in preparation for childbearing. It also makes fat cells stick together, contributing to the dimply effect of cellulite.

But those lumps are also signs of an unhealthy lifestyle. Having cellulite doesn't mean you're fat—just toxic. You can greatly minimize cellulite with a few simple lifestyle changes:

* Drink three liters of water with lemon juice throughout the day to prevent water retention and flush the liver—a culprit in cellulite formation.

* Cut fried and processed foods and pass on the Big Macs. These foods ultimately interfere with blood circulation and lymph drainage. Sluggish circulation and drainage prevent sufficient waste and toxin elimination. Lymph builds up and makes cellulite appear worse.

* Go green. Fill up on these cellulite-busting vegetables: celery, kale, broccoli, brussels sprouts, parsley, green peppers, and root veggies like turnips and parsnips. These foods nourish the liver and have a detoxifying effect on the body. Asparagus is a great diuretic to help prevent water retention.

* Eat apples. An apple a day can keep cellulite away. The pectin found in apples (and carrots) is an important phytochemical that strengthens the immune and detoxification systems of the body.

* Exercise. It helps by increasing lymph flow. In addition, weight lifting builds more muscle, making the skin overlying your hips and thighs more taut. The tighter your skin, the less obvious the cellulite is.

2 You *Are* a Sugar Addict

The biggest reason people get fat is sugar. I work with overweight clients who tell me all the time, "I don't really like sweets." After surveying their diets, I see that they're loaded with bread, yogurt, and cereals—all foods that are laced with hidden sugars. They don't eat plain oatmeal, for example; they eat a bowl of apple cinnamon oatmeal containing eleven grams of sugar. If this sounds like your dietary habits, trust me, you're addicted to sugar, whether you realize it or not. I know I was.

In This Chapter:

* *Sugar overload and weight gain*
* *Sugar addiction*
* *Hidden sugars*
* *How sugar kills*

When I was younger, I was hooked on daily candy, Pop-Tarts, sugary cereal, and soda. Sugar became my number-one coping mechanism; eating it was part of my routine. I liked the instant high I felt, and I looked forward to all my processed goodies throughout the day. I especially loved anything that combined bread and sugar—you know, like doughnuts and cupcakes. Because of my addiction to sugar, I was hyperactive in school and had learning disabilities. But they all cleared up when I decreased sugar in my diet. I now know sugar for what it is: poison to your system.

I've said it to my clients a million times: Sugar is the devil. It has zero nutritional value and weakens your immune system. It throws off your metabolic functions and is highly addictive.

Years ago, I came across the book *Sugar Blues,* in which author William Dufty spelled out his theory that sugar is a drug, not a food. He called the sugar pick-me-up "mortgaged energy," because "more and more nutrients are required from deep in the body in the attempt to rectify the imbalance" in your system. Once I read that book, I never thought about sugar the same way again. His book led me to design my five-days-on, two-days-off plan, in which you cut out sugar for five days in a row and let your brain and body start functioning normally. You'll learn more about this in chapter 5.

But let me say this now: You will be so excited when you see how fast you lose weight on this plan—and how wonderful you'll feel—after you kick your sugar habit. A lot of experts want you to believe that grazing on small amounts of sugar daily is fine. I'm here to tell you it's not! Sugar is the most damaging ingredient in the American diet. It's making you fat and sick!

Sugar, Sugar Everywhere

Sugar is the leading food additive in the U.S. food supply and is making us a nation of sugar junkies. You're fed sugar in almost every product from childbirth on. It's in practically everything you eat now. In fact, the average American downs thirty teaspoons of added sugar daily! That's 480 nutritionally empty calories of added sugar every day. As a nation, we're pushing maximum density. Headlines call it "an epidemic of obesity." It's no coincidence that this epidemic has progressed in step with our sugar consumption.

Refined sugar is technically sucrose, or common table sugar. The other sugars you need to be aware of include dextrose (corn sugar), fructose (fruit sugar), maltose (malt sugar), and lactose (milk sugar).

Refined white sugar was once scarce and extremely expensive, a luxury only the wealthy could afford. Early devotees termed it "white gold," using it only to sweeten the most costly of dishes. The earliest attempts at sugar refining began in the fourth century, in Persia and ancient Arabia, where it was extracted from sugarcane and made into large, golden-brown blocks. Early sugar was less refined—it actually had nutrients in it—and wasn't made with the nasty chemicals found in today's counterpart.

You hear sugar advertised as a "natural" food because it's made from the natural ingredients in sugarcane and sugar beets. Unfortunately, many people have come to equate *natural* with *healthy*. There's nothing natural about sucrose! Ninety percent of the original source (sugarcane or sugar beets) has been removed. The natural brownish color is lightened by chemical bleaching. What's left is white sugar, stripped of all its minerals and vitamins. Cocaine, too, could be advertised as "made from natural ingredients." The coca leaf from which it is made is as natural as sugarcane. Both leaf and cane yield similar products—a white crystalline powder with horrible effects.

Sugar isn't just bad nutrition; it's health-damaging nutrition. Here's what I mean: When sugar is found in natural foods and plants (such as apples, berries, or even sugarcane), it comes in a package with the vitamins, minerals, and enzymes needed for its complete digestion. When it's found in sugar packets or in candy or in the disaster known as high-fructose corn syrup, it contains nothing of any good. The body actually has to borrow from its stores of nutrients in order to process it. Sugar literally eats up the nutrients your body needs to stay healthy. This depresses your immune system, and that's why sugar can make you so sick.

Your Brain on Sugar

When you eat refined sugar, it goes straight to your intestines, bypassing any chemical breakdown in your body. From the intestines, it's absorbed right into the bloodstream. Your blood glucose level spikes fast. Your brain registers this sugar hit with a drug-like reaction. Sugar triggers the release of the same natural brain opioids released when shooting heroin, which are associated with positive feelings such as pleasure, energy, and euphoria. That release makes most people feel good, but it makes sugar-addicted people feel absolutely high. And when sugar is taken away, you get the same withdrawal signs, including "the shakes" and changes in brain chemistry, as those caused by withdrawal from heroin, nicotine, or booze. As drugs do, sugar stimulates the reward pathways of the brain.

When you're addicted to sugar, you need more to feel better. Your life starts being focused on getting a sugar fix. And by the way, when I talk about sugar, I don't just mean candy and cookies. I'm also talking about carbohydrates that are quickly converted to sugar, such as bagels, breads, croutons, rolls, crackers, and more. Their rapid conversion to sugar causes a corresponding hike in insulin. High insulin prevents the breakdown of body fat.

When you're on sugar, the brain signals insulin to rush in and hold down the sugar. Glucose levels then plummet. The adrenal glands have to step in to release fat-producing cortisol to get them back up again. Blood sugar levels crash. You feel tired, irritable, jumpy, and mentally sluggish. The body's specially balanced mechanisms are just not designed to cope with these sudden, rapid changes in sugar levels.

There is a built-in biological reason that we crave sugary foods. Back when we were foraging through the forest for any little nut or berry as cave dwellers, we developed a genetic predisposition for certain foods. Generally, the fruits and vegetables that tasted sweet were healthy, so we ate them. Foods that tasted bitter were often poisonous. Our instinct for sweetness ensured that we got the nutrients necessary to survive. Of course, our caveman ancestors never ate sugar as pure white sugar. The sweetness of nature for them came embedded in fruits and other plants. In today's world, processed foods loaded with sugar are a common staple. So if you want to get thin, repeat after me: Eat like a cave woman.

Sure, I'll admit that alcohol and drug addictions seem like worse threats—but are they? When you find out how sugar is linked to disease and depression, you will think again. If you think you're sick now, here are the horrifying facts of what's to come if you keep eating sugar.

Sugar Makes You Fat

Excess sugar wreaks havoc on every organ in the body. Initially, it's stored in the liver in the form of glycogen. But the liver can hold only so much before it inflates like a balloon. When the liver's storage capacity gets maxed out, glycogen is expelled in the form of fatty acids. These travel to every part of the body and lodge themselves in our fatty areas: the belly, hips and butt, breasts, and thighs. After these areas are filled, the remaining fatty acids get dealt out to the major organs, including the heart and kidneys. Fat nestles there, releasing toxic chemicals that damage arteries, blood vessels, and organs. Sugar also causes a sluggish metabolism—not to mention the worthless calories it adds. When calories go up, so does your weight.

Not only does ordinary sugar make you fat, so does another common additive in processed foods: high-fructose corn syrup. Made from cornstarch, high-fructose corn syrup is found in everything from cereals to protein bars to breads. The big problem with this crap is that it's quickly metabolized as fat and prevents the body from knowing it's full. This is why you can sit down with a box of cookies or chips and eat them until they're gone.

Fructose as a naturally occurring fruit sugar—found, for example, in an apple—is absolutely fine because it's surrounded with healthful nutrients, phytochemicals, and fiber. But when fructose is extracted, refined, and made into a liquid sweetener, it's a poison. Sucrose and high-fructose corn syrup are nightmares, and people eat too much of both.

Sugar Grows Cancer

Does it feel like everywhere you turn, someone else is getting cancer? Or maybe that someone is you. One in three people will get cancer in their lifetime. I don't like those odds! My mother fought it with chemotherapy, and I promise you, it is one of the nastiest diseases that you can deal with. We all have cells in our bodies that, under favorable conditions, could mutate into cancer anytime. One of those conditions is a high-sugar diet.

Cancer cells multiply rapidly. This process requires a lot of energy. To get enough energy, cancer cells supercharge themselves with glucose. Cancer cells love sugar. Sugar makes tumors grow. You can help stop cells from mutating into cancer through diet and exercise. The most important dietary change you can make will be to greatly decrease the toxin sugar in your diet.

Sugar, of course, jacks up insulin levels. Insulin problems—too much or too little—go far, far beyond diabetes. Insulin stimulates cell growth. Unfortunately, cancer cells have six to ten times the number of insulin receptors—molecules that grab on to the hormone—as normal cells. So if extra insulin hits a preexisting cancer cell, it makes a bad thing deadly. For cancer, insulin is like pouring gasoline on a fire. All this contributes to a greater risk of cancer, because cancer cells thrive when sugar is available.

Here's a partial list of cancers you may be at greater risk of because of sugar:

* ***Breast cancer.*** The chance of a woman having breast cancer at some point during her life is about one in eight. It is the second leading cause of cancer death in women, after lung cancer. A study conducted in Italy and published in 2006 in *Annals of Oncology* found that breast cancer rates coincided with high sugar consumption in thousands of women. The more sugar women ate, the higher their risk. Another study showed that women who are overweight and have high blood sugar tend to develop a very aggressive type of breast cancer that usually kills. This research was published in 2003 in *Cancer Epidemiology Biomarkers & Prevention.* Is eating too much sugar worth losing your breasts, or your life?

* ***Pancreatic cancer.*** This is the most lethal of cancers, killing about thirty thousand Americans each year. It usually spreads rapidly and is seldom detected in the early stages. High insulin levels are thought to trigger this horrible cancer.

* ***Colon cancer.*** This is the third most common cancer among men and women, and has a higher death rate than both breast and prostate cancers. In a study from Harvard, people who ate sugar-infused junk like breads, cereals, cookies, cakes, and other sweets made with white flour were nearly three times more likely to get colon cancer than those who rarely ate those foods. The link between diet and colon cancer is just too strong to ignore.

* ***Stomach cancer.*** Pure white sugar without fiber, minerals, and vitamins irritates the lining of the stomach and intestinal walls. This increases the risk of stomach cancer, a deadly cancer that kills six out of ten patients.

* ***Endometrial cancer.*** This is the most common female gynecological cancer in the United States. A risk factor is estrogen. We talked about how estrogen dominance makes you fat, but it may also increase the risk of getting this cancer. Look at your diet: If it's high in processed foods, you're in trouble.

This is just the short list of cancers that may be caused in part by sugar. Cancer is a painful disease, and chemo is something you should want to avoid in life at all costs. It harms your body, and you may never fully recover. If this information doesn't make you want to give up sugar, I don't know what will!

Sugar Gives You Wrinkles

Sugar makes you fat and may increase your risk of cancer. Guess what else? It ages your skin and causes wrinkles.

In a process called glycation, eating sugar attacks collagen and elastin, both key proteins that make your skin look young. Glycation makes them less elastic and more brittle so they break. Your skin can't snap back. That's when fine lines and wrinkles appear, and they don't go away. You're stuck with them.

But it gets worse. Collagen and elastin start to mutate, creating harmful new molecules called advanced glycation end products (AGEs). These build up and cause further inflammation and damage to your collagen and elastin. Sugar actively ages you.

Ditching sugar will make you look and feel ten years younger. Save your money on expensive plastic surgery remedies to look more youthful, and put it into healthier, whole foods and treats.

LOW-BLOOD-SUGAR BLUES

OD ON SUGAR, and you set yourself up for, ironically, low blood sugar or hypoglycemia. The symptoms hit a few hours after a sugar binge: dizziness, weakness, tremors, sweating, even heart palpitations. Because sugar is broken down so fast, the rush of insulin quickly depletes the glucose, and there's nothing left in reserve. You're in a state of low blood sugar. About one in every one thousand Americans is walking around with it. It's not only diabetics who need to be concerned with hypoglycemia. It's everyone. Low blood sugar causes:

* Weight gain
* Slow metabolism
* Irritability and depression
* Constant cravings
* Mental confusion

* Recurrent yeast infections
* Chronic fatigue
* Migraines
* Damage to vital organs
* Coma and death (in uncontrolled diabetes)

Sugar Kills Your Immune System

Sugar wrecks your immune system. Eating just a few teaspoons of sugar can cripple the capacity of certain white blood cells called neutrophils to engulf and destroy bacteria. Neutrophils make up 65 percent of the total white blood cells in circulation. With neutrophils out of commission, you're vulnerable to developing colds, flu, infections—even chronic fatigue syndrome (CFS). With CFS, you feel inexplicably run-down and unrefreshed by sleep. You will not have the energy for intense workouts. And you will want to eat more. You're as healthy as your immune system. Give up sugar!

Sugar Makes You Stupid

Our brains are very sensitive and react to quick chemical changes within the body, including those caused by too much sugar. Researchers now report that people who have even slightly elevated blood sugar concentrations also have short-term memory impairment. Researchers at the Nathan S. Kline Institute for Psychiatric Research in Orangeburg, New York, tested thirty people without any history of memory problems. They found that when volunteers were given an infusion of pure sugar, they couldn't recall the details of a brief story that had been read to them. Recall was worse if a person didn't metabolize sugar well—which is usually the case if you eat too much sugar.

What was going on? Scientists think that high-sugar diets disturb blood sugar metabolism. When blood sugar is out of whack, or you have trouble metabolizing sugar, this shrinks memory areas in the brain.

You can change the course at any time by eating differently. Don't be stupid; don't get stupid. Get off sugar!

To Avoid Sugar, You Have to Know Where It Hides

Okay, you understand that sugar is a major weight gainer, disease causer, and chronic fatiguer. Now let's talk about how it's cleverly hidden in virtually everything we eat, especially packaged and processed foods, from breads and crackers to soups, sauces, and entrées—and even diet foods and low-fat foods. But first, here's my guideline for sugar:

Choose foods with five grams of sugar per serving or less. The body doesn't register anything five grams and under, so that is optimal.

Popular breakfast cereals are among the worst offenders. For example, start your day with a supposedly good-for-you cup of raisin bran, and you've ingested twenty grams of sugar—about the same as gobbling nine Hershey's Kisses. Special K's Fruit and Yogurt cereal, another product disguised as healthy, contains eleven grams of sugar. As for hot cereals, a packet of Quaker sweetened instant oatmeal—like Maple & Brown Sugar or Apples & Cinnamon—includes some thirteen grams of sugar, almost all of it table sugar. Then, when you add a cup of nonfat milk, you are adding fourteen more grams of sugar in the form of lactose. Don't eat this crap! Only get the plain oats that have no sugar. You can add cinnamon, blueberries, and Truvia (a stevia-based sweetener) for sweetening.

Of course, children's cereals are nothing more than candy. A 2008 analysis by *Consumer Reports* found that eleven popular breakfast cereals contain at least 40 percent sugar by weight. That's at least as much sugar as you'd get in a glazed doughnut at the doughnut shop. The analysis was based on a study published in the *Journal of the American Dietetics Association.*

As for the bagel you grab every morning, unless you get whole wheat or multigrain, your bagel is essentially three to five 1-ounce slices of nutritionally dead white bread. Some specialty bagels, such as Dutch apple & raisin bagels, contain thirty-three grams of sugar. That's the same amount you get in a piece of chocolate cake!

Sugar hides in foods under clever names like beet sugar, brown sugar, cane sugar, confectioners' sugar, corn syrup, dextrose, fructose, high-fructose corn syrup, invert sugar, lactose, maltodextrin, maltitol (a sugar alcohol), mannitol (a sugar alcohol), sorbitol (a sugar alcohol), sucrose, and turbinado sugar. These sugars are in everything from protein bars and shakes to breads and dairy. Don't waste your time looking at the ingredients on the label. You're just going to be overwhelmed. Eat only the foods that have five grams or under per serving, and you will be fine.

ARE YOU A SUGAR ADDICT?

Sugar addiction is serious. To see if you're really hooked, take this questionnaire. Answer yes or no to the questions below, and be as honest as you can.

1. Do you snack frequently on sweet foods or drink sweet beverages between meals?

2. Do you often feel shaky, weak, or irritable after eating sugary foods?

3. Do you eat sugary desserts most days of the week?

4. Would you describe yourself as chronically tired most days of the week?

5. Do you usually put sugar in coffee or tea?

6. Do you use sweet condiments (jams, jellies, syrups, and the like) daily?

7. At parties, do you gravitate toward the sweets?

8. When you were a kid, did your parents give you sweets for being good?

9. After eating sweets, do you feel euphoric, only to have your mood plunge afterward?

10. When you get cravings, are they mostly for bread or sweets?

11. Do you suffer from frequent headaches?

12. Do you usually grab a doughnut or bagel for breakfast?

13. Do you drink soft drinks almost daily?

14. When you go to the snack counter at the movies, do you usually buy candy?

15. If you order an alcoholic beverage, is it usually something sweet like a piña colada or frozen margarita?

If you answered yes to three or more questions, the chances are that you are a sugar addict.

Fat-Free, Sugar-Heavy

One of the biggest places sugar hides is in fat-free foods like cakes, cookies, ice cream, salad dressings, and snacks. These foods often contain more sugar (and sometimes more calories!) than the regular versions. Why? Manufacturers took the fat out of food and boosted the sugar to give it flavor. A SnackWell devil's food cookie has fifty calories and no fat. A Keebler Soft Batch cookie has eighty calories and 3.5 grams of fat. Which cookie has more sugar? The SnackWell with seven grams, compared with five grams in the Keebler. Remember, fat doesn't make you fat, sugar does.

One of the cruelest hoaxes played on us involves "diet" products. If you want to lose weight, you could enjoy a healthy, low-calorie meal like a grilled chicken salad with low-cal dressing. Or you could chow down on high-fructose corn syrup, yogurt-flavored coating, partially defatted peanut flour, honey, corn syrup, and the other ingredients in some of the popular nutrition bars out there. Everything in these products blocks fat-burning hormones!

Sugar is found not only in things that are sweet, which we know have sugar, but also in other processed foods that don't taste particularly sweet. That includes ketchup, canned beans, barbecue sauce, and spaghetti sauce. I could go on and on—but I think you get the picture. Sugar is hidden everywhere.

Stop the Sugar Blues!

Trust me, sugar is affecting your body in a very bad way, and you've got to kick the habit. Indulging in sugar-laden foods sets you up for getting fat and not feeling well. Remember, blood sugar spikes, followed by blood sugar drops, lead to tiredness, irritability, sugar cravings, weight gain, and eventually all sorts of terrible health problems. Here's how to be sugar-free:

* Get rid of sugar-free juices, sodas, and treats. They cause sugar cravings. A diet soda actually triggers your brain to grab for chips or other junk foods.

* Don't allow sugar in your clean products like water, tea, or coffee. These are necessities in many of our lives and should remain completely sugar-free. Many people lose weight by not adding sugar to foods.

* Go to the fridge and pantry and rid your life of simple sugar items including (but not limited to): candy, cookies, cakes, sodas, fat-free products, and products made from these products. It's impossible to keep unhealthy foods in the house without indulging. If you try to keep them, you will fail and hate yourself for it. Treat meals should be bought, indulged in, and any leftovers thrown away immediately. Be strong. You won't crave sugar as much once the cycle is broken, and you can use treat meals to indulge. Just don't keep sugary stuff in the house.

* Buy apples, pears, berries, and citrus foods instead. They're lower in simple sugars and calories, and provide vitamins you won't find in items like candy and sodas. Citrus fruits and apples, in particular, help your body burn fat. The more whole fruit you eat, the less processed sugar you will crave. It won't send your blood sugar levels on a roller-coaster ride, and the fiber in the fruit will fill you up.

* Buy Truvia, a low-cal natural sweetener sold in grocery stores, drugstores, and online.

* Exercise regularly. Exercise kills cravings for junk, as well as making you a fat-burning machine throughout the day. Just twenty minutes a day of rigorous physical activity brings the rush of endorphins your brain wants to replace a sugar rush. In fact, when you feel a craving coming on, immediately step outside for a walk, take the stairs, or hop on the treadmill. Lunch workouts are a great midday way to kill the cravings. Pretty soon, you'll want the endorphins from the workout more than the cheesecake.

* Graze on healthy snacks throughout the day. The traditional three-meal-a-day diet hasn't done much for sugar addicts. The full feeling after a meal turns to hunger in a matter of three or four hours, leaving you susceptible to sugar cravings. Make healthy snacks accessible all throughout the day and use them to keep your stomach full.

* Drink lots of water. A craving is often a sign of plain dehydration, not a cry for food. So carry a bottle of water or iced herbal tea to combat those sugar attacks. Drinking two to three liters of water a day burns fifty to seventy-five additional calories, and speeds up your metabolism.

* Cut back on caffeine. Plain and simple, caffeine can cause a drop in blood sugar levels that leads to fat storing. Switch to herbal tea, if possible, or have no more than two cups of coffee a day.

* Stick to my eating plan. It will help you kick your sugar addiction. Here's a preview of what's in store: Monday through Friday, do not eat refined sugar or products that contain over five grams per serving. On my plan, you'll do this for five days—the time it takes to break the chemical addiction in your brain. On the weekend, you'll get to indulge in two treat meals. This schedule of eating will help you naturally need less sugar to feel satisfied. In two weeks' time, you'll notice that the quantities you used to consume are now too rich for you. This is your body's natural response mechanism and a sign that it's starting to balance itself.

By following just three of the above tips, you will lose weight without even walking into a gym. Choose what you can live with and start losing for longer and start living stronger.

3 Three Organs That Make You Fat or Skinny

The third reason you're getting fat is your organs: an overworked liver, a sluggish thyroid, and exhausted adrenals. These organs rule your metabolism—the rate your body burns off food calories. When they're not working up to par, it's very hard to build muscle or burn fat. This means you won't get all the benefits from eating right or exercising.

In This Chapter:

* *Detoxify your liver*
* *Thyroid and metabolism*
* *Avoid adrenal burnout*

I am so obsessed with keeping these three organs clean that I eat detox foods *and* take supplements. Trainers in my gym constantly compare notes on how to flush these organs, knowing that when working well, they will speed up the metabolism big-time. So if you want to get thin, make sure you do everything you can to clean these three organs. Like everything else, you can do this through diet and lifestyle.

If You Live in America, Your Liver Is Overworked

The liver makes proteins that regulate blood clotting, neutralizes toxins in the blood, produces immune agents to fight infection, generates bile to help digest fats, and stores glucose for when you need energy. The liver is basically the metabolic factory of the entire body. It can make you a fat-storing machine or a fat-burning machine, depending on how you treat it.

Your liver burns fat in several ways. For one thing, it manufactures bile acids. These are like laundry detergent. They break down the cheese fries you threw down last night. Bile acids also switch on the activity of brown fat—a calorie incinerator that burns calories instead of storing them. In addition, bile acids carry excess fat to the small intestines for disposal. If your diet is high in fiber from fruits, veggies, and whole grains, this unwanted fat is then washed from the body through your bowel.

Your liver's job is also to detoxify everything you eat, drink, swallow, smoke, rub into your skin, or otherwise work into your bloodstream. Almost every substance found in your body or put in your body, including hormones, chemicals, bacteria, viruses, fungi, and parasites, is filtered through the liver for removal. So think of the liver as your body's garbage disposal. It works nonstop to clean up and remove junk from your body.

And like a garbage disposal, the liver is vulnerable to overload. When that overload happens, it can't detoxify all the junk that comes its way. Nor can it do a good job of breaking down proteins, carbs, and fats. The body then starts poisoning itself. This is often what's happening to people who are chronically sick with headaches, inflammatory diseases, and skin disorders, such as psoriasis and acne. Toxins that can't be processed by the liver escape into the bloodstream, wiping out the immune system. The result is autoimmune disorders like fibromyalgia, chronic fatigue syndrome, lupus, and arthritis in which the body turns on itself.

Do You Have a Sick Liver?

You may think that, as long as you're not knocking back a bottle of booze every night, your liver will take care of itself. Don't kid yourself. For years, doctors thought pretty much the same thing, only testing blood levels for telltale signs of liver disease such as hepatitis or cirrhosis.

Things are different now. We have many more toxins in this country than the rest of the world. Third-world residents have healthier diets and livers than we do. They don't add all the chemicals to their foods, and they don't pump up their meats with hormones—which is in part why their citizens are thinner. But in this country, more people than ever are sick and heavy as a result. And so health professionals have started to take a much closer look at the liver.

Here are some telltale signs of a sick liver:

* Weight gain, especially around the belly

* Cellulite

* Bloating

* Allergies

* Gluten intolerance

* Indigestion

* Constipation

* High blood pressure

* High cholesterol

* Hormone imbalance

* Hypoglycemia (low blood sugar)

* Fatigue

* Depression

* Mood swings

* Yeast overgrowth

* Skin disorders

* Sleeplessness

* Brain confusion

* Bad breath

* Itchiness

* Stool that is discolored (should be dark brown)

ORGAN MAINTENANCE—GET YOUNGER!

LIKE MANY WOMEN, I was once convinced that anti-aging and a beautiful body could be achieved only through exercising, diet, and keeping up with endless skin-care "breakthroughs." But then I learned that there is a far more powerful force than all those things combined: organ health.

The liver and other organs get worn down by toxins in our diet and the environment; by consuming too much fat, sugar, caffeine, alcohol, and nicotine; by the ultraviolet rays of the sun; and by the many other physical and emotional stresses to which we subject our bodies. The cumulative effect is aging.

This is why, if you spend all your money on facials, moisturizers, laser wrinkle removal, makeup, and clothes, you'll never feel or look as good as you would if you spent more time on detoxing and taking care of your liver. Follow the advice here, stimulating your liver, thyroid, and adrenals to stay healthy, and you'll turn back the clock.

If you're overweight or suffer from any of the above symptoms, then the detox foods on my program are a must for you. The great news is that the liver is resourceful and repairable. It can be restored and rejuvenated. You've just got to take steps to cleanse and detoxify it.

Two main advantages here: First, your body will burn fat more efficiently—you'll lose weight. Second, a healthy liver will make you less vulnerable to dietary indulgences. You won't have to panic when you indulge yourself with your treat meals like a cheeseburger or sundae, because as long as you quickly get back to my five-day eat-clean plan, those treats will burn themselves off on their own.

Trainers know this. We're notorious for our treat meals. They never seem to affect us because we eat so clean *most* of the time. For example, I eat a multitude of all the foods my body needs to run well and burn fat, with the understanding I'm going to indulge in my comfort meals on the weekend. When you eat this way, instead of stressing the liver out daily with junk, it will recover fast.

Getting Fatter? Thyroid Problem!

Have you noticed your pants getting tighter when you're trying to lose weight? That the scale is going up for no apparent reason? Why are you gaining weight?

One reason may be your thyroid, another key organ of metabolism. The thyroid gland can make you either love your body or want to hide in baggy sweatpants. It's your body's metabolic regulator. It controls metabolism by secreting two hormones that control how fast the body burns calories and uses energy. If your thyroid secretes too little hormone, you have hypothyroidism, or underactive thyroid. All of this slows down all your bodily functions. Hypothyroidism leaves you tired and makes it more difficult to burn calories. Because everything is slowed, the body will demand quick energy all the time in carbohydrate cravings—which is why low thyroid sufferers crave refined carbs like breads, pastas, cereal, crackers, cakes, muffins, rice cakes, cookies, juice, alcohol, ice cream, and so forth. Simply put, if your thyroid isn't working to stimulate your metabolism, it is very tough to get thin. Just by living in this country and consuming processed food, you probably have an underactive thyroid. There's one more thing: I call the thyroid the beauty gland because if it's working right, it makes your hair and nails healthy.

Signs of a Sluggish Thyroid

Doctors have trouble diagnosing hypothyroidism. This is because it shows up as a variety of symptoms that are often identical to those you have if your life is hectic or that might occur normally as you get older. For example:

* Weight gain

* Cravings for refined carbs

* Fatigue (often due to malnutrition, since the thyroid controls vitamin absorption)

* Loss of appetite

* Foggy thinking

* Inability to tolerate cold

* A slow heart rate

* Painful menstrual periods

* Muscle weakness

* Muscle cramps

* Dry, scaly skin

* Poor fingernail growth (the thyroid controls hair and nail growth; a faulty thyroid is a disaster for hair and nails)

* Hair loss

* Migraines

* Hoarseness

* Itchy skin

* Depression

* Dizziness

* Heart palpitations

* Weird burning sensations in the body

* Constipation

* Difficulty concentrating

* Bags under your eyes

* Yellow bumps on your eyelids

In general, your risk for hypothyroidism increases with age, particularly for women over thirty-four. Some experts suggest that up to 25 percent of all women will eventually develop a thyroid problem.

If you have hypothyroidism, don't just rely on your doctor to write a prescription. Taking thyroid medication blocks your own body's ability to produce the hormone on its own. That is never good, and you will be on it for life with greater problems. You can balance your thyroid naturally through food and exercise.

Your Wiped-Out Adrenal Glands

The adrenal glands produce the hormones adrenaline, norepinephrine, DHEA, and cortisol (the fat-storing hormone I talked about in chapter 1). All of these hormones help your body naturally cope with stress. They do this by triggering the release of sugar from the liver and muscles into the blood as an instant fuel source.

DHEA is a sex hormone and natural fat burner. I call it the mother of all hormones because most of our other sex hormones are derived from it, primarily estrogen and testosterone. This important muscle-building and fat-burning hormone declines with age, which makes it even harder to stay thin and fit. You want to do everything you can to keep your adrenal glands healthy so they can produce this amazing hormone.

Are You Headed for Adrenal Burnout?

For everything they do, your adrenals take a lot of abuse. We batter our adrenals with bad nutrition, lack of sleep, smoking, drinking, and medication abuse. But the greatest enemy of the adrenals is our reliance on caffeine-containing products like coffee and sodas.

If you're consuming more than two cups of coffee a day, you are at risk of overworking the adrenal glands. I know this from research as well as from experience. Trainers are the worst adrenal abusers. Because of their schedules—sporadic hard work over a long day—they easily get hooked on pick-me-ups like coffee. After a month or two, taking in so much caffeine noticeably exhausts them.

Caffeine is also found in dietary supplements, namely those containing caffeine-rich herbs like guarana, yerba mate, or green tea. In a study funded by the Agricultural Research Service (ARS) in Beltsville, Maryland, scientists analyzed fifty-three dietary supplements—predominantly weight-loss and sports-nutrition products with at least one caffeine-containing ingredient. Approximately half of the tested products contained the caffeine equivalent of up to two cups of coffee per day!

When the adrenals get overworked by caffeine and other factors, they eventually can't produce hormones in sufficient amounts, or can't utilize the hormones they do produce. Basically, the adrenals get wiped out. This condition is called adrenal exhaustion, and it makes you a slow metabolizer, tired all the time, and generally unwell.

So look at the chart below, and analyze how much caffeine you are truly taking in each day. Cut your caffeine intake drastically, and after a couple of weeks you will feel better. Every time you want a coffee, drink a bottle of cold water. It is nature's energizer.

CAFFEINE CONTENT IN BEVERAGES AND DRUGS

BEVERAGES AND FOODS	RANGE (MG)
Coffee	
Brewed, 5 oz. cup	*115–180*
Starbucks brewed coffee (Grande), 16 oz.	*320*
Espresso, 1 oz.	*30–90*
Instant, 5 oz. cup	*65*
Tea, 5 oz. cup	*40*

Soft Drinks (12 oz. can)	Range (mg)
Jolt Cola	72
Mountain Dew	55
Diet Mountain Dew	55
Coca-Cola, Diet Coke	34
Dr Pepper	43
Diet Dr Pepper	44
Pepsi-Cola	39
Diet Pepsi	37

Energy Drinks	Range (mg)
Rockstar Energy Drink, 8 oz.	80
Red Bull, 8 oz.	80
Red Bull, Sugarfree, 8 oz.	80
Rip It, 8 oz.	100
Monster Energy, 16 oz.	160

Over-the-Counter Drugs	Range (mg)
NoDoz maximum strength, 1 tablet	200
Vivarin, 1 tablet	200
Excedrin (extra strength), 2 tablets	130
Anacin (maximum strength), 2 tablets	64

Sources: Company websites or scientific articles

Key symptoms of adrenal exhaustion include:

* Weight gain, especially around the belly

* Weakness

* Blemishes (when you're under stress, cortisol causes more pore-clogging oil to be produced)

* Insomnia (caused by cortisol being elevated at night)

* Lethargy

* Dizziness

* Headaches

* Memory problems

* Food cravings

* Poor immunity

* Allergies

* Blood sugar imbalances

* Premature aging

Cure Organ Dysfunction and Burn Fat Like Crazy

Give your liver, thyroid, and adrenals what they need, avoid giving them what they don't need, and they will reciprocate by burning fat. Your weight will come off almost automatically. This is all pretty simple, too. Really, all it takes to cleanse and detoxify is swapping out most of the bad stuff for the good stuff. To avoid getting fat and breeding cancer and other diseases, give your organs the recommended daily amounts of vitamins, minerals, and nutrients through a combination of food and a carefully planned program of natural supplements. Here are some things you can start doing now:

* Eat detox foods daily. Many foods have organ-protective properties. My nutrition plan is built around detox foods, including apricots, artichokes, beets, blueberries, and green leafy vegetables. With my plan, you'll learn how to build these foods into your diet.

* Drink two to three liters of pure water a day. It's worth the extra trips to the bathroom! Water is vital for keeping your system clean. It helps with detoxification and assists bile acids in flushing out toxins. Add some lemon juice to it. Remember, this combo is a natural fat metabolizer and can burn fifty to seventy-five calories a day. Also, if you drink this much water daily, you can boost your metabolism by as much as 30 percent.

* Get as much organic food as you possibly can. Ever heard of organochlorines? Most people haven't. They're awful chemicals found in pesticides (which are sprayed all over fruits and vegetables). With these chemicals in your body, you'll burn fat more slowly than normal. To reduce your risk, grab organic produce. It contains fewer toxins and will make life easier for your liver.

* Supplement with liver-friendly herbs. I take a liver-cleanse supplement that contains milk thistle. This herb functions as an antioxidant in the liver. Antioxidants fight free radicals, the big villains behind disease and aging. Other top liver healers include licorice root, skullcap, red clover blossom, and slippery elm bark. You can find these supplements at any health-food or vitamin store.

* Increase your fiber. High-fiber foods such as fruits, veggies, and whole grains remove toxins from the body. Make sure you eat between twenty-five and thirty-five grams a day for healthy digestion and liver health. An example of what this looks like daily is a cup of oatmeal, an apple, a cup of mixed berries, a salad with veggies, and a cup of frozen or fresh spinach.

* Add whey protein to your diet. Whey protein is a high-quality protein powder and available as a protein supplement. It suppresses the buildup of fat in the liver, plus revs up fat-burning activity. Any low-sugar or sugar-free whey protein shake is an excellent supplement to your diet.

* Get enough B vitamins. Choline, vitamin B_6, folic acid, and vitamin B_{12} are among the lipotropic nutrients, meaning they're involved in the movement of fats. You can get vitamin B from green leafy vegetables, oranges, brown rice, oats, wheat germ, fish, shellfish, eggs, and poultry, as well as from a daily multivitamin tablet.

* Eat plenty of vitamin-C-rich foods, including citrus fruits, berries, kiwi fruits, parsley, watercress, and peppers.

* Include in your diet magnesium-rich foods like whole grains, green leafy vegetables, sunflower and sesame seeds, almonds, and wheat germ.

* Regular exercise. There's no getting out of doing some sort of physical activity if you want to keep your metabolism high. Exercise has a positive effect on all body systems.

Avoid the Organ Destroyers

An important part of a rejuvenation program for your organs is easing off organ destroyers. These are toxic substances that increase your appetite, slow your metabolism, interfere with your ability to burn fat, and mess up your system. Sure, there are some toxins in the environment you can't control. But there are a whole lot more you can, and they're found in the food supply. Here's some stuff you should eat less of, or give up altogether:

* Alcohol. Cut back on your alcohol consumption, or stop completely. If you're a social drinker or someone who has a drink more than once a week, you'd better know that this habit is making you soft and chubby. Not only because it adds sugar and calories, but also because it prevents the liver from metabolizing fat properly. Enjoy alcohol as part of a treat meal and limit it to once per week.

* Fatty meats. Unless it's a treat meal, don't let deep-fried, smoked, salt-cured (think jerkies), or fatty foods pass your lips. The liver has to work overtime to break these foods down. They're high in saturated fat, which increases the risk of a fatty liver. These foods also put unnecessary stress on the adrenals.

* Excessive amounts of milk and other dairy products. Sickening high levels of artificial hormones, antibiotics, and other toxins are found in dairy products. The liver must go into overdrive to try to eliminate them. One of the most toxic substances in the world—dioxin—is found in dairy products. Dioxin can cause cancer in humans. Even minuscule doses can deal a stunning blow to the immune system. Unless milk is part of your treat meals, stay away from it. Don't worry about getting enough calcium and vitamin D. You will get plenty with the natural foods I recommend.

* Junk foods. Ditch junk, fried, and fast foods, unless they're a part of a treat meal. Eating junk food and fake foods will never get you to where you want to be. They stress the liver by making it work too hard at removing the chemicals, additives, and fat in these foods.

* Refined carbs. These include white bread, white flour, white pasta, white rice, and, of course, white sugar—they're all just empty calories with no real nutritional value, and are so bad for you. Even in moderation, they all disrupt liver functioning. Your liver has to work too hard to process sugar and sugary foods. Sugar, in particular, robs your body of valuable nutrients like zinc. You need zinc; it helps the liver burn fat.

* Acetaminophen products, such as Tylenol. The leading cause of acute liver failure in the United States today is not alcohol or hepatitis but overdoses of acetaminophen. If you take it regularly, your liver will not metabolize fat efficiently.

* Prescription drugs. Drugs affect liver function and cause weight gain. Medicine is nothing more than a bunch of chemicals that stress the liver and keep it from burning fat. After working with me, it's amazing how many of my clients are able to go off or greatly reduce their medications.

* Antihistamines. These drugs can interfere with thyroid functioning.

* Fluoride in tap water. Fluoride blocks iodine receptors in the thyroid gland. Iodine, a mineral key to thyroid health, can't get access to cells. This halts hormone production and causes hypothyroidism. Buy jugs of natural mineral water or get a water filter.

* Sugars and refined carbohydrates. Sugar breaks down so fast that it shocks the liver. These substances also deplete magnesium, throw all hormones out of whack, and make you fat.

* Substances such as caffeine, tobacco, and, again, alcohol. They rob the body of nutrients required by your organs, so cutting your intake of these will help your stress levels and decrease your fat.

* Artificial sweeteners. These include sugar alcohols, aspartame, saccharine, sucralose, and others. These nasty substances aggravate cortisol and wipe out adrenals.

WAS TOM CRUISE REALLY CRAZY?

MANY OF US WERE SHOCKED at how fanatical Tom Cruise got when discussing drugs as a business in this nation, but he makes some very solid points. He has basically pointed out the damaging effects that drugs have on the body.

We are a drug-dependent society, and the dealers are the doctors and pharmaceutical companies. The medical industry is keeping us addicted, polluted, and toxic. For proof: Almost half of Americans take at least one prescription drug every day; one in six take three or more daily. Today, prescription drugs have become interwoven with the very notion of what constitutes health. Pills are expected to make us thin and happy, wake us up, put us to sleep, improve all kinds of performance, and lengthen our lives.

Yet pills can be damaging to your health and your spirit. Many drugs cause a drastic change in your body chemistry, as well as prevent your body's ability to naturally produce the substance it's lacking and being medicated for. You get hooked for life and need more and more to feel okay. One drug dependence almost always leads to another.

I've seen this with my own clients. They start by taking popular sleep aids to sleep, drinking coffee to wake up, then progressing to a mood stabilizer or anti-anxiety drug because they feel stressed. Most of them started off with just the sleep aid! Do you see how the body gets thrown off? Never work against your body's delicate balancing system with meds unless you absolutely must. Think less medication, more motivation, and think of food and exercise as powerful medicine. Indeed, they're more powerful than any drug you'll ever take. If you eat more nutrients, cut down on sugar, and maintain a regular exercise program, you won't need as many drugs, or any at all! You won't suffer much fatigue or depression or other lifestyle ills, because you will constantly have endorphins and health-sustaining nutrients running through your system. The body is a self-regulating machine. If you follow my program, your body will naturally balance itself. Of course, always talk to your doctor before beginning any program or decreasing medications, because many produce strong withdrawal symptoms that can be dangerous, or the medications may be critical for your health.

Now you understand how the liver, thyroid, and adrenals are keys to a healthy, fat-burning metabolism—and a healthy, energetic lifestyle. Take care of them if you want a thin body for the rest of your life—and lots of energy to go along with it. Keeping these organs in peak condition is easy to do, and you will feel so much better for it. Put my strategies into play, and they'll increase your overall health and fitness while giving you a beautiful, thin body and your best, sexiest size.

Now it's time to talk about how.

Part 2

THIS IS HOW YOU EAT TO GET HOT AND HEALTHY

4 Add to Lose

My 2-Week Jump Start

What if I told you that I'm not going to take away any of the crappy foods you're currently eating? That's right! My clients are ecstatic when I share this news. For the first two weeks, my plan actually adds food to your existing diet. So stop worrying about deprivation and start getting excited about nutrition. Think of my food plan as the first "nondiet" diet you've ever been on. I don't care if you're eating fried chicken, pizza, or ice cream every night of the week right now. I know that sounds crazy, but there is a method to my madness.

In This Chapter:

* Add in fat-burning foods without changing your diet

* Supplement your diet to maximize your results

* Subtract foods that cause sensitivities

The first part of my eating plan lasts two weeks. All you do during those two weeks is add in some specific foods every day. When you do so, you will rapidly change your body chemistry and satisfy your physical and emotional hungers. I stumbled on this add-food philosophy quite by accident. I always ask my new clients to give me a seven-day food journal before we even start our exercise program. As I mentioned earlier, most of their daily entries were pretty similar—and disturbing. They'd start off with no breakfast or a high-calorie breakfast, followed by long stretches of food deprivation and topped off with a huge meal for dinner because they were starving to death.

Also, important nutrients were missing from their diets. In fact, everyone who was chunky and sluggish was totally nutrient-deprived. I decided to experiment by adding several nutrient-rich foods into their existing diet every day. They were shocked to see their weight going down even before they started training with me. These results intrigued me enough to research and find a tremendous amount of data that supported what was really happening. What I found out was that adding nutrient-rich foods into your diet will naturally curb your cravings for sugary and fatty foods. Your body starts correcting itself with these nutrients, and you will not crave junk food nearly as much. In fact, expect your cravings and desire for junk food *to greatly decrease in fourteen days.*

Here's how the first two weeks will work.

Every Day for the Next Fourteen Days, Add in the Following Foods

EGGS (2 DAILY)

I love eggs because they are such a great fat-burning food. They supply a nutrient called lecithin, which breaks down fat in the body. A study in the *Journal of the American College of Nutrition* compared overweight women who ate bagels for breakfast with overweight women who ate two eggs. The latter group lost 65 percent more weight and had an 83 percent decrease in waist circumference.

Eating eggs also curbs your appetite. You'll feel fuller a lot longer. Eggs can be hard-boiled, soft-boiled, poached, or scrambled, but without added fat.

> *Quick Tip:* Boil a whole carton of eggs, peel them, and place two each in six ziplock bags. Shake in salt and pepper, then stick the bags in your fridge. You'll have a portable snack for the whole week!

Oatmeal (1 cup daily)

Oatmeal is another of my favorite fat-burning foods. It's one of the healthy carbs and is less likely to be deposited as body fat than many other carb sources. It digests slowly, which means that your body gets a steady stream—rather than a tide—of energy as carbohydrates gradually flow into your bloodstream. And it fills you up and kills your cravings.

Oatmeal also keeps insulin levels low and steady to prevent weight gain. Additionally, it's a whole grain, which means it's full of soluble fiber—the good stuff that carries fat out of your body. Oatmeal also contains the energizing—and stress-lowering—B vitamin family, which helps transform carbs into usable energy.

> *Quick Tip:* I keep packets of instant oatmeal on me at all times. When I go to a Starbucks or any other eatery, I ask for a cup of hot water to prepare the oatmeal, and I eat it down in a few bites. I look at my instant oatmeal as a vitamin, not a meal.

Hormone-Balancing, Detox Vegetables (2–3 cups daily)

Stuff yourself with these! Vegetables are nature's fat burners. They fill you up without filling you out because they're loaded with fiber and water. You can eat all you want and lose weight. Start by adding in two to three cups of vegetables to your daily meals. This is as easy as having a salad loaded with your favorite veggies and adding some steamed veggies at dinner.

The vegetables I recommend on my two-week plan include artichokes, asparagus, broccoli, brussels sprouts, cabbage, carrots, cauliflower, celery, collard greens, cucumbers, eggplant, endive, garlic, green beans, kale, lettuce (all varieties), mushrooms, mustard greens, onions, parsley, peppers (all varieties), radishes, scallions, spinach, summer squash, Swiss chard, tomatoes, turnip greens, watercress, yellow wax beans, and zucchini. All of these veggies have a hormone-balancing, detoxifying, and fat-burning effect on the body. As a result, your body uses them for nutrition rather than storing them in fat cells.

> *Quick Tip:* I don't love vegetables, so I sneak them into my regular meals. I add a handful of fresh spinach to my fruit shake in the morning (the fruit cuts the bitterness of the greens). Also, I keep broccoli in the freezer at work; every day I microwave a cup for one minute twenty-five seconds and just gobble it down in a couple of bites. This is another one of my "vitamins."

Fresh Fruit (2 servings is 2 whole fruits)

Controlling your sweet tooth is less about willpower and more about support foods like fruit. Just adding more fruit to your diet will cut down on your desire for sweets. So begin trading your daily bread or candy fix for fresh fruit, like watermelon wedges or mango slices. Your taste buds will start to anticipate the naturally sweet taste of the fruit. Fruit is also a great source of soluble fiber that takes up a lot of space in your stomach, digests slowly, and fills you up.

Loading up your diet with fruit will help your weight drop. Overweight women who ate two hundred calories a day in apples and pears while eating a healthy diet lost more weight than women who didn't eat fruit at all, according to a study conducted by Brazilian researchers at the Universidade Federal do Amazonas. And like the veggies listed above, fruit has a balancing, detoxifying, and fat-burning effect on the body. All of this makes it an ideal food for weight loss.

Fruits to include are apples, apricots, bananas (underripe), berries (all varieties), cherries, citrus fruits (all varieties), kiwi, guava, mango, melon (all varieties), papaya, pear, peach, pineapple, plum, pomegranate, and watermelon. A serving generally equals one piece of raw fruit or one cup of chopped fresh fruit.

> *Quick Tip:* Always eat whole fruit, never juice. Use one fruit in your morning shake, then eat an easy, portable fruit like a pear or apple in the afternoon.

Water and Lemon Juice

Drinking lots of water with lemon juice—two to three liters a day—will activate the burning off of stored fat in your body. Why? Water with lemon juice is a bile thinner. This means it helps bile do a better job of processing fat.

Water and lemon juice also prevent cravings—which means fewer snack attacks during the day. We often confuse simple thirst with a craving for food. Sipping water fills your stomach and ensures that you're not grazing on junk when you really just need to replenish H_2O. And with more water in your system, expect to feel more energetic and get a clearer complexion.

> *Quick Tip:* Wake up in the morning and drink a bottle of water along with your morning coffee. This will hydrate you, and you can use the restroom before work!

WHEY PROTEIN SHAKE (8-OUNCE SERVING DAILY)

Whey protein powder mixed with eight ounces of water is a terrific detoxifier. Whey is also quickly digested and put to use by the body. It's a natural fat burner, and it improves insulin levels, making whey one of your best allies for losing excess pounds and controlling your weight. And it stimulates the production of an antioxidant called glutathione, which supports fat burning by your liver. There's more to the astonishing facts about whey. It has the highest levels of branched-chain amino acids (BCAAs) of any protein source. BCAA content is important because these amino acids are an integral part of muscle development. Whey is thus a terrific muscle builder. Each day, have a low-sugar whey isolate protein powder from any vitamin shop or drugstore. Add a scoop to eight ounces of water and enjoy.

> *Quick Tip:* Supplement with extra BCAAs (see page 64) and flaxseed oil fortified with omega-3s to really boost your body's fat-burning potential. You can buy these items at a vitamin or health-food store, as well as at a Whole Foods market.

HERBAL TEAS

To satisfy oral fixations (most late-night snacks are really about oral compulsions), have one packet of decaffeinated green tea with one packet of herbal fruit tea every evening. Green tea contains L-theanine, a chemical that increases dopamine and serotonin in the brain, two chemicals that regulate appetite, mood, energy, and cravings. It also contains compounds that block fat storage. The herbal fruit tea gives green tea a delicious flavor.

> *Quick Tip:* Drink this tea at the time of night in which you are most likely to have cravings. For me, it's 9 PM in front of the TV.

Why This Plan Works

When I first tell my clients about this two-week jump start, some of them are worried that they are going to overeat and won't lose weight. Nothing could be farther from the truth!

This plan is specifically designed to control your appetite and cravings while balancing your body chemistry. And it is the attention to this single purpose that produces results. Your cravings stay quiet, and you have the energy for your workouts.

Imagine what it will feel like to have even more control over the way you look and feel by being able to simply add in a few foods to your diet. As you adjust to these additions, the compulsion to pig out on the higher-calorie stuff diminishes. Within two weeks, you'll be eating less junk food automatically—and loving healthy food more. And before long, you'll have a body that you'll be proud of.

Add in Supplements!

Unfortunately, nutrient-deprived bodies need assistance to get strong and balanced. There are some supplements I swear by and that will really aid in your weight-loss journey. I call these the good food additives because they boost what naturally occurs in a healthy, athletic body. Regular use of multivitamins and other key supplements helps support muscle development, helps curb cravings, and promotes good health. Here are the supplements I love—and why you should start adding them to your diet now.

Multi-Vitamin-Mineral Tablet

A broad-spectrum multi-vitamin-mineral supplement is a great way to ensure that your basic, but indispensable, nutritional needs are met. Multiple vitamins and minerals also help you get certain nutrients that support fat loss. For example:

* *Magnesium.* This mineral plays a central role in the secretion and action of insulin. A deficiency here makes control of blood sugar levels impossible, deactivates enzymes that accelerate metabolism, and triggers cravings.

* *Zinc.* This mineral builds human growth hormone. Low zinc levels lead to low levels of testosterone. Being low in zinc can also interfere with thyroid hormone

production, leading to a lowered metabolic rate and making it harder to drop body fat.

* *B vitamins.* Many of the B vitamins, such as niacin (and niacinamide) and biotin, play important roles in energy production and fat loss.

* *Fat-soluble vitamins.* These include vitamins A, D, E, and K. They're called fat-soluble because they're absorbed by fat cells and not by water. If these vitamins are in short supply, you could start craving fatty foods—which makes supplementation a good idea.

Take one multi-vitamin-mineral pill a day with food.

OMEGA-3 FATTY ACIDS

Contrary to what you've heard, you should *not* cut fat from your diet. In fact, you should be putting the right kinds of fat back into your diet. This will help you lose even more weight.

Among the best fats to add in are omega-3 fatty acids. They help you control your weight, increase exercise performance, block inflammation and pain, enhance the efficiency of leptin (a hormone that tells your body you're full), prevent depression, and protect joints. Omega-3s also tame your appetite. That means you'll lose pounds more easily!

There are three kinds of omega-3s: DHA, EPA, and ALA. DHA and EPA are the omega-3s found in fish. ALA is found in non-animal sources like flaxseed, walnuts, and some vegetable oils. Both varieties offer benefits.

To make sure you're getting enough of these amazing fats, take one to three grams of omega-3 supplements daily with food.

VITAMIN C

Everyone thinks vitamin C is a cold remedy. But guess what? It's a fat remedy. Vitamin C has a stabilizing effect on your adrenal glands, and this helps control the level of fat-storing hormones like cortisol in your body. When your adrenal glands overproduce cortisol in response to stress, the glands eventually become exhausted, and you feel the same way. Cravings for sweet or salty snacks, or for coffee or other stimulant beverages, may be a side effect. Adrenals love vitamin C. In essence, this vitamin feeds these glands and enables them to function more optimally despite extra demands.

Here's a fact that blew me away: People who increase vitamin C by five hundred milligrams a day burn nearly 40 percent more fat during exercise and 30 percent more fat while resting. Even though my plan includes plenty of high–vitamin C foods, I suggest taking a vitamin C supplement that supplies at least five hundred milligrams of this nutrient. I recommend a formula that contains Ester-C. This is a patented, non-acidic, natural form of vitamin C that allows cells to effectively absorb high levels, yet doesn't upset the stomach and is gentler on your digestive system than other forms of vitamin C.

BCAAs and Free-Form Amino Acids

I suggest to my clients that they supplement with free-form amino acids, available in capsules, powders, or liquid. I have been taking aminos for years. They are so important for beauty, de-aging, and weight loss. They work by building collagen to make your skin beautiful, removing liver toxins to help you burn fat, and increasing growth hormone for muscle tone.

You'll want to choose a formulation that contains a complete and balanced blend of aminos, specifically including isoleucine, leucine, and valine (the BCAAs). BCAAs greatly aid in how well your body maintains muscle. Make sure that the amino acid glutamine is included in the formulation, too. Glutamine is involved in more metabolic processes than any other amino. It prevents muscle breakdown and boosts your immune system. Glutamine also plays a role in the regulation of body weight, as well as the metabolism of sugars and fats. For dosage, follow the manufacturer's recommendations.

Creatine

This supplement raises your metabolic rate slightly. Since your metabolic rate represents the number of calories you normally burn each day, boosting it with creatine can help you burn more body fat over the long haul. Another way it enhances fat loss is by increasing muscle strength. You're able to work out harder for greater fat loss.

Be sure to purchase creatine ethyl ester HCL instead of regular creatine monohydrate. Creatine ethyl ester HCL is better absorbed and will not cause bloating. Follow the manufacturer's guidelines for dosage.

CLA (CONJUGATED LINOLEIC ACID)

A fatty acid derived from sunflower oil and found in dairy products and red meat, CLA both blocks fat storage and prompts cells to dump the fat they're already holding. This supplement also helps you develop muscle as well as lose fat. Take one to three grams of CLA with breakfast, lunch, and dinner.

All these supplements can be found in a health-food store like Vitamin Shoppe or GNC, organic markets, and some drugstores.

Dealing with Food Sensitivities: When to Subtract Foods

It seems that everybody I talk to these days has some sort of food intolerance or allergy, including myself. Today, twelve million Americans, or 4 percent of the population, have some form of a food allergy, according to the Food Allergy & Anaphylaxis Network.

I ate a ton of bread growing up, and even now when I feel like treating myself, I gravitate toward bread products like pretzels, crackers, and croissants. However, in my late thirties, I noticed that I would get a terrible burning pain in my stomach after consuming bread. This aggravating condition was later diagnosed as gluten intolerance. Now, why would this happen to me out of nowhere, especially since I don't eat much bread now?

Researchers don't know for sure why food allergies are increasing. Some experts say it's our modern lifestyle. People are stressed out, and stress inflames the gut. The body reacts to this by producing antibodies in an allergic response. Also, the ingredients in all the processed foods we eat may trigger allergic reactions.

With allergies on the rise, there may be some foods you'll want to *subtract* from your diet at the same time you're adding in foods for the next two weeks. This is important: Food allergies and food intolerances can make you fat, bloated, and metabolically inefficient. For these reasons, I recommend to my clients that they pay attention to foods they might be sensitive to—and begin to subtract them from their diets.

Some foods to watch include dairy products and wheat. If dairy products are a problem, you may have lactose intolerance. People with this condition lack the enzyme to break down lactose in cow's milk and milk-based products.

If you're lactose-intolerant, you have options. You can subtract dairy products from your diet altogether, get your calcium from a supplement or foods like greens and almonds, and make up the protein by increasing your intake of lean meats, eggs, or vegetarian sources of protein. Or you can try some of the products on the market targeted toward the lactose-intolerant, including milk that's lactose-free. Or use lactase pills, which can be taken before eating dairy products.

Another common food intolerance is gluten intolerance, which is what I have. It's the inability to digest or break down gluten, a protein that's found in wheat, barley, and rye. This problem is on the rise due to the overprocessing and overuse of wheat in too many everyday products and junk foods. If you have to subtract gluten and wheat foods from your diet, replace them with gluten-free products. For baking, you can use rice, corn, and potato flour in place of ordinary flour.

If you notice any symptoms, keep track of the amount and type of foods you eat and any bad physical reactions you have afterward. This will clue you in to possible sensitivities.

Do not skip my two-week jump start. It's designed to start changing your body chemistry and metabolism for weight loss. By following these guidelines for just two weeks, you'll start losing weight. Your body is a perfect machine and wants to work for you. You just have to give it the right fuel and it will! Now let's get into the details of what to do next, after these important two weeks are up.

5 Deprivation Doesn't Work

My 5 + 2 Food Plan

In This Chapter:

* Hormone balancers and detox foods
* Meal planning
* Where do calories fit in?
* Enjoy your treat meals

You've just completed fourteen days of adding specific foods into your diet. These foods have begun the process of changing your body chemistry, recharging your metabolism, and managing your cravings. You no longer have to add them in, but they will be incorporated as part of your meal choices from here on out. If you hop on the scales after fourteen days, expect to see fewer pounds. Even your clothes should feel looser. View these changes as positive transformations. Your body is no longer in "fat mode." It's in a fat-burning mode!

Now it's time to transition to the next stage: what I call my 5 + 2 Food Plan. This plan says: Eat clean, healthy foods for five days (Monday through Friday), then enjoy two treat meals on the weekend. Treat meals can and should include your favorite foods.

I'm the only fitness professional who allows two treat meals. After working with countless clients, I found that one treat meal was not enough to stay on track long-term. Clients felt literally cheated out of one of life's greatest pleasures, and they started slipping up all through the week. Not until I added the second treat meal did everyone start responding in phenomenal ways.

No desserts. No candy. No cocktails. No snacking. No enjoyment from food whatsoever—no wonder we hate dieting so much. It's associated with total deprivation! My 5 + 2 Plan is not a diet. Diets are associated with total deprivation! Deprivation does not work. I actually get resentful and start sabotaging myself if I have to say no too many times. This is the case with most people. Denying yourself food to lose weight isn't necessary. The harder you try to stick to a diet, giving up your favorite foods, the more likely you are to fail, and the more you're likely to crave those foods. You starve, sacrifice, and suffer with your weight, and all the while your emotions go up and down like a roller coaster. Usually, you'll cave in and end up overeating. Many of you end up heavier than before you started.

There are only two rules with my 5 + 2 Plan: You have to eat clean for five days in a row, and when you have your treat meals, those meals can't exceed fifteen hundred calories each. That's a lot of food! This approach is an easy, sustainable way to get thin and be healthier. It guides you into making small, simple changes in your eating habits, your attitudes, and your mental and emotional state. It also continues to rebalance your body chemistry, break your sugar addiction, and boost your metabolism so that getting thin is easy, natural—and enjoyable. Your body becomes further primed to burning fat all day long. So get excited about your new journey. You'll love the freedom. You'll love the way you feel about yourself. And you'll love the results.

Eat Clean in a Dirty World

Now that you've added foods in for the past two weeks—and you're getting used to a better diet—it's time to get serious and eat "clean." Eating clean means eating foods that:

* Burn fat

* Build lean muscle

* Balance your hormones

* Detox your body

You're probably thinking, *Wow, can food do all that?* Yes! Each of us is a body factory. We grow, think, feel, heal, move, breathe, and reproduce ourselves—by making natural chemicals, including hormones and endorphins. And like any other factory, we need certain raw materials for this manufacturing process. These raw materials are nutrients—and we get them from food.

Most people these days have no clue how to eat right. And many "experts" have made dieting so complicated and unrealistic that people tend to give up. In fact, diets have a 98 percent failure rate! Well, I'm going to make it simple for you. Remember, no complicated diets here. I'm going to show you how to eat clean in a dirty world. Once you get the hang of it, it's easy to do, and you'll never want to make dirty eating a lifestyle again. With this in mind, I've created a list of clean foods you will eat on my 5 + 2 Plan: All of them are hormone balancers and detox foods.

Hormone-Balancing Detox Proteins: Eat Four 4-Ounce Servings a Day

FISH AND SHELLFISH

Protein, in general, is a great fat burner because it speeds up your metabolism. And fish and shellfish are among the best sources of protein. As hormone balancers, they're hard to beat. Fish—particularly sources like salmon that are high in omega-3 fatty acids—has a beneficial effect on leptin levels, which means it helps suppress your appetite. Seafood also helps alter fat distribution on the body, increases testosterone production, and is high in zinc to help build human growth hormone (HGH) for a leaner body. Shellfish is high in iodine, which speeds up the metabolic rate.

Selections

Clams	Lobster
Cod	Mackerel
Flounder	Monkfish
Grouper	Orange roughy
Haddock	Oysters
Halibut	Perch

Pollack

Red snapper

Salmon, wild

Sardines, water-packed

Scallops

Shark

Shrimp

Sole

Tilapia

Trout

Tuna (fresh or low-sodium canned)

Whitefish

LEAN POULTRY (CHICKEN AND TURKEY)

Like all proteins, poultry is high in amino acids. Amino acids buffer cortisol release and help increase testosterone production, making poultry a great hormone-balancing choice. Plus, it's low in fat. Always choose free-range poultry, if available.

Selections

Chicken breasts, skinless

Cornish hen, skinless

Turkey breast, skinless

LEAN MEAT

You might be surprised to learn that I allow meat, including red meat. Why? Because it can actually aid with weight loss. Red meat, in particular, yields the highest, most efficient rate of growth for muscle (more muscle means more fat burning). Red meat also supplies nutrients that are key to metabolism: vitamin B, iron, creatine, amino acids, and zinc. Lean meats help balance hormones because they're high in the mineral chromium, which helps stabilize blood sugar. Make sure you choose lean cuts like those listed below. Also, select products that are grass-fed. A word of advice: Enjoy meat occasionally, like twice a week, and preferably after you've started your cardio/resistance-training program.

Selections

Flank steak

Sirloin

Tenderloin

Pork tenderloin

Pork rib chops

Pork roast

Lamb roast

Lamb chops

Leg of lamb

LOW-FAT DAIRY FOODS

Dairy foods are important, too, because they accelerate fat loss, particularly in the tummy, by reversing a fat-forming hormonal process. I support low-fat, low-calorie cheeses in moderation (see my list below). By far, my favorite dairy protein is low-fat cottage cheese. It supplies casein and the amino acid glutamine to burn fat and assist in recovery after exercise. Greek-style yogurt is a good choice, too; it has less sugar than conventional yogurts. Try to combine dairy with a veggie or fruit to fill you up and add flavor to your snacks or meals.

I would rather that you not drink cow's milk. It is high in milk sugar, and milk sugar is fat forming. Don't worry about not getting enough calcium and vitamin D if you don't drink milk or eat other dairy products. You can get plenty of calcium from other sources. Nondairy sources of calcium include almonds, broccoli, beans, tofu, figs, bok choy, and green leafy veggies; nondairy sources of vitamin D are cold-water fish (for example, salmon, trout, herring, sardines, mackerel) and sunlight.

Selections

Greek-style yogurt

Low-calorie cheeses (Brie, Camembert, Fontina, low-fat cheddar, Edam, feta, goat, Limburger, and part-skim mozzarella)

Low-fat cottage cheese

Almond milk

Low-fat ricotta cheese

EGGS

Eggs are a superb form of well-absorbed protein and a great detox food. They contain lecithin, which promotes healthy liver function, thereby helping the body burn fat.

BEANS AND OTHER LEGUMES

These foods are exceptional hormone balancers and detox foods, plus a great source of protein. Also, they normalize insulin levels and help keep your blood sugar steady throughout the day. They're high in fiber, too, which stimulates the release of appetite-suppressing hormones. Garbanzo beans, lentils (including lentil soups), red beans, and soybeans have specific detox properties.

Selections

Adzuki beans	Lentils
Bean soups	Lentil soups
Black beans	Lima beans
Black-eyed peas	Navy beans
Broad beans	Pinto beans
Fava beans	Red beans
Garbanzos	Soybeans
Great northern beans	Split peas
Kidney beans	White beans

WHEY PROTEIN

Whey protein is one of the most nutritious proteins you can choose. It contains branched-chain amino acids (BCAAs), which are critical in building lean muscle. Whey is a natural detoxifier, too, promoting the health of the liver to flush impurities from the body. You started using whey protein in your diet during my two-week jump start; continue supplementing your diet with this important protein.

FITTING IN YOUR PROTEIN

* Have at least one 4-ounce serving of protein at each major meal—breakfast, lunch, and dinner—and another serving as part of a snack. This will provide your four daily servings of protein. Eat a variety of proteins from my list, including vegetarian proteins.

* If you eat dairy foods, limit them to one of your protein servings per day.

* As for eggs, two a day equals one protein serving. I suggest that you try to eat two eggs each day.

* A daily scoop of whey protein counts as one protein serving. You can make a great shake by combining fruit, water, and whey protein.

FAT-BURNING FACT: PROTEIN

IN MOST AMERICANS' DIETS, protein makes up about 15 percent of total calories. According to research from the University of Washington, when dieters bumped their protein intake to 30 percent (and reduced their fat to 20 percent), they were eleven pounds lighter on average, even though half their calories still came from carbs. They also reported feeling more satisfied with less food. Higher protein sparks the production of glucose in the small intestine. This increase, sensed in the liver, and relayed to appetite control centers of the brain, suppresses the appetite. Protein is an amazing appetite suppressant.

Source: American Journal of Clinical Nutrition

Hormone-Balancing/Detox Carbohydrates

The carbohydrates on my plan are slow-digesting carbs. They break down gradually in the body and don't spike insulin and blood sugar levels—which means they won't make you fat. Also, they provide steady energy and replenish muscle glycogen for strength and power. These good carbs come from plants and include foods such as whole grains, vegetables, most fruits, dark nutty breads, legumes, and beans.

These foods are also high in fiber. Fiber is either insoluble or soluble. Both types help make you thin. Insoluble fiber in whole grains, bran, nuts, and vegetables serves to move fat and extra calories out of your body. Soluble fiber found in oats, fruit skins, and flaxseed forms a gel in the intestine, keeping you full longer and slowing the release of glucose from food into the bloodstream. This keeps you from storing fat. So if you want to be lean and healthy, eat both types of fiber. Here's a closer look at the carbs on my program.

Hormone-Balancing/Detox Vegetables: Eat 3 Cups a Day

VEGETABLES

Vegetables contain slow-digesting carbohydrates that help normalize blood sugar levels. They also supply many vital nutrients, and their enzymes work as natural detox agents. Beets help purify the blood, asparagus relieves water weight gain, and artichokes enhance liver function, to name just a few benefits. Certain veggies like broccoli, spinach, sweet potatoes, and tomatoes are considered superfoods because they saturate the body with health-building nutrients. Incorporating more vegetables in your diet keeps your body functioning properly and burning fat.

Selections

Alfalfa	Kale
Artichokes	Kelp and other edible seaweeds
Artichoke hearts	Kohlrabi
Asparagus	Leeks
Beets	Lettuce, all varieties
Beet greens	Mushrooms
Broccoli	Mustard greens
Broccoli sprouts	Okra
Brussels sprouts	Onion
Cabbage	Parsley
Carrots	Parsnips
Cauliflower	Pea pods
Celery	Peas
Chiles	Peppers, all varieties
Cilantro	Potatoes
Collard greens	Pumpkin
Corn	Radishes
Cucumbers	Rhubarb
Dandelion greens	Rutabaga
Eggplant	Scallions
Endive	Spinach
Fennel	Summer squash
Garlic	Sweet potato
Green beans	Swiss chard
Jicama	Tomato

Turnips

Turnip greens

Watercress

Winter squash (acorn, butternut, et cetera)

Yams

Yellow wax beans

Zucchini

Hormone-Balancing/Detox Fruits: Eat 2 Whole Fruits a Day

Fruits contain slow-digesting carbohydrates for stabilized insulin levels, and they're also rich in fat-fighting fiber. Apples, melons, lemons, pineapple, and other detox fruits nourish and detoxify the body for more efficient fat burning. Be sure to eat citrus fruits, too; they're loaded with fat-burning vitamin C.

Selections

Acerola cherries

Apples

Apricots

Bananas, underripe

Blackberries

Blueberries

Cantaloupe

Casaba

Cherries

Cranberries

Currants

Dates

Figs

Grapes

Kiwi

Kumquats

Grapefruit

Guava

Honeydew

Lemon

Lime

Mango

Oranges

Papaya

Peaches

Pears

Pineapple

Plums

Pomegranate

Prunes

Raisins

Raspberries

Strawberries

Tangelos

Tangerines

Watermelon

Hormone-Balancing/Detox Grains: Eat Two 1-Cup Servings a Day

Grains are high in fiber, which provides bulk, stimulates the release of appetite-suppressing hormones, and increases the time it takes for food to move through your intestinal system, meaning that fewer calories are left to be stored as fat. Grains such as bran and quinoa are human growth hormone (HGH) building blocks. Grains also enhance normal insulin secretion.

Selections

Barley	Oat bran
Bran	Quinoa
Brown rice	Rye
Buckwheat	Spelt
Bulgur wheat	Wheat germ
Cornmeal	Whole-grain products (dark nutty
Millet	breads, crackers, pita bread,
Oats	tortillas, and so on)

Quick Tips for Carbs:

Eat like a diabetic! Always try to combine carbs with protein in a meal to slow the digestion of the carbohydrate food. For example: grilled salmon with a sweet potato; scrambled eggs with oatmeal; or whole-grain crackers and low-fat cheddar cheese. Carbs eaten alone can digest rapidly into sugar; this spikes insulin, increases appetite, and slows metabolism.

Mix small portions of starchier carbs, such as whole-grain pasta or brown rice, with larger portions of low-calorie veggies like green beans, broccoli, mushrooms, onions, bell peppers, or cauliflower. You can save hundreds of calories over a week.

Eat canned beans. They're quick to prepare and can easily be packed for lunch.

Eat carbs earlier in the day. Carbs eaten less than three hours before going to bed can cause an overnight buildup of fat, decrease the production of human growth hormone, and cause cortisol (a fat-gainer chemical) levels to rise.

Hormone-Balancing/Detox Fats (1 serving = 2 tablespoons of oil, ¼ cup of nuts or seeds, or ¼ avocado)

You need some fat in your diet for energy, beautiful skin, and the production of testosterone. My plan emphasizes clean fats over bad fats. Among the clean fats are omega-3 fats, found in fish and flaxseed. These fats create an environment in your body that balances insulin levels. Balanced insulin helps you get thin and stay thin. Omega-3 fats also trigger hormones to burn more fat. Other good fats are found in olive oil, avocados, walnuts and other nuts, and seeds. These foods contain monounsaturated fats, which help regulate blood sugar and protect the heart and the immune system.

Bad fats cause you to be fat. They include saturated fats found in whole milk and tropical oils. Beef contains saturated fat, too, but it's fine to include some beef in your diet as long as you choose lean cuts.

Trans fats are the worst of the bad fats. These are human-made fats listed as hydrogenated oil or hydrogenated vegetable oil on food labels. Avoid them at all costs. They break down muscle and weaken your immune system.

The amount of bad fat in your diet is very much related to weight gain. Your body turns bad fats into body fat much faster than good fats. What's more, bad fats slow down metabolism by as much as 25 percent. So if you eat a lot of bad fats, you will see the pounds pile on quickly, particularly in areas like your hips, thighs, belly, and around major organs.

Selections

Almonds	Olive oil
Almond butter (raw)	Peanut butter
Avocado	Pecans
Brazil nuts	Pumpkin seeds
Butter	Sesame seeds
Flaxseeds	Sunflower seeds
Flaxseed oil	Walnuts
Hazelnuts	Walnut oil

I WANT TO SHARE with you that I was once a vegan. My reason for choosing that lifestyle was the horrific and cruel treatment of animals in our society. I am totally against factory farming and have hopes that our country will strongly legislate against the cruelty being perpetrated by these soulless industries. Even so, research and my own personal experience support the fact that the body needs some lean meat for optimal performance and weight loss. Of course, not eating animal products is a personal choice. If you do eat animal products, I strongly advise that you always buy hormone-free, cruelty-free, and free-range foods.

FITTING FAT IN

A daily fat serving equals two tablespoons of clean oils, nut butters, or nuts or seeds; and a quarter avocado.

Quick Tips for Fats:

Prepare foods by roasting, baking, broiling, steaming, or grilling—without added fat.

Use olive oil spray to give foods a hint of fat.

Remove skin and visible fat prior to cooking.

Make your own salad dressings using balsamic vinegar and olive oil. For one serving, mix 2 teaspoons of olive oil with 2 tablespoons of balsamic vinegar. This gives you 75 calories in a serving. Try to stick to no more than 75 calories a serving with any salad dressing. When eating out, ask for dressing on the side and order a balsamic or low-fat dressing.

Spread peanut or raw almond butter on toast rather than butter. Raw almond butter, as opposed to roasted, is higher in nutrients and a more effective fat burner. The protein in these nut butters, combined with the carbs in your toast, will slow digestion and make you feel full. Nut butters are also good fats with hormone-balancing benefits.

Use seasonings more, and butter less.

Use low-fat salad dressings and low-fat mayonnaise as condiments.

Cook with extra-lean ground turkey in place of ground beef. (My recipes offer delicious ways to substitute.)

Beverages

Reminder: Always try to drink three liters of water daily, particularly combined with a dash of lemon juice. This will help for a number of reasons. First of all, it will aid in flushing the body of toxins and impurities. Drinking water with meals will help to fill you up so you will be less apt to eat as much of the bad foods. As an added benefit, water helps promote fat burning. Continue to have decaf green tea and herbal fruit tea in the evening.

DON'T GO LOW-CARB!

CARBOHYDRATES ENERGIZE your body and brain. So if you cut back on carbs too much, you will feel horrible. Low-carb diets deplete your body of glycogen, the muscle fuel it makes from carb-rich foods. Strange things start happening to your body when it's deprived of glycogen. Without it, your body makes a less efficient fuel from fat. That fuel is called ketones. Ketones are nasty. They give you bad breath, make you feel dizzy and tired, and make your system slow to a crawl; some research shows they may also cause acid buildup in the bloodstream—which can be lethal. Low-carb eating lowers brain levels of serotonin, a chemical critical to controlling depression and anxiety. So you want to make sure you're eating enough carbs.

Portion Control

You've also got to master portion control to get thin. That means learning what a real serving size is—and how many of those portions you can eat and still lose weight. Unfortunately, hardly anyone knows this these days because everything is "supersized." A good example is pasta in a restaurant. When you get your order, your plate probably holds four cups of pasta. That's technically eight servings! You're about to eat fourteen hundred calories in one sitting. There goes your entire day.

If you don't want to use a food scale, measuring cups, or measuring spoons, you can use your hand as a measuring guide. The hand method works like this:

* Eat a salad the size of both hands put together. This equals a little more than a cup of greens.

* Eat fish, poultry, and lean meats the size and thickness of the center of your palm. This equates to four ounces of meat.

* Eat a serving of hard cheese, salad dressing, oil, nut butter, nuts, or seeds the size of two thumbs. This measurement equals two tablespoons or, in the case of cheese, one ounce.

* Eat a serving of veggies, chopped fresh fruit, milk, low-fat cottage cheese, or Greek-style yogurt the size of your fist. The same goes for cereal, rice, pasta, cooked grains, and cooked beans or legumes. A fist-size portion is the same as one cup.

Eat 5 Times a Day

Eating five times a day will stabilize your blood sugar. If your blood sugar gets high, your body will overproduce insulin, and insulin makes your body store fat. Your five meals should include breakfast, lunch, dinner, a midmorning snack, and a midafternoon snack. You will lose weight more quickly if you eat on a schedule like this, rather than only one or two meals.

Quick Tip: To make this easy, cook and prepare food in bulk ahead of time. Put your food in Tupperware containers or ziplock bags right after you prepare it and when you get home from the grocery store. Some great "bagged" foods include:

Two boiled eggs and a little salt and pepper

Several celery sticks spread with nut butter

Apples with low-fat string cheese

Chicken or turkey breasts with brown rice and broccoli

Instant oatmeal packets (no sugar added)

I prepare my foods like this and then just grab the bags when I'm on the road or leave the house. Invest in a freezer bag, too, in which you can carry and store a whole day's worth of food, then microwave it. Expensive delivery diets do this. You can buy these bags at any major chain store like Kmart, Wal-Mart, or Target.

Creating Your Meals

Using the food selection guidelines I've outlined, your meals during the week will look something like these.

BREAKFAST

Protein (2 eggs, for example)

Grain (1 cup of oatmeal, for example)

Fruit (1 cup of fresh berries, for example)

SNACK

Protein shake (scoop of whey mixed with water and fresh fruit, for example)

LUNCH

4 ounces of protein (baked chicken breast, for example)

1 cup of a vegetable or 1 baked sweet potato

SNACK

¼ avocado or 1 cup of chopped fresh veggies, for example

DINNER

      4 ounces of protein (sirloin steak, for example)

      Grain (1 cup of brown rice, for example)

      Vegetable (1 cup of steamed broccoli, for example)

This sample menu gives you the right complement of foods for the day: four proteins, three veggies, two grains, two fruits, and one fat. For more ideas, there is a month's worth of sample meals in appendix A, and several include the recipes that go along with my eating program.

By eating hormone balancers and detox foods and giving yourself a break from refined flour, sugar, and other junk, your body can shed up to ten pounds of excess water weight, and your energy soars. All of these foods support the body's natural ability to rid itself of toxins, help you get thin, improve your digestion, and keep you from feeling bloated and congested. Choose these foods, build your meals around them, and you'll totally change the way you look and feel for the rest of your life.

Enjoy 2 Treat Meals on the Weekend

After you've eaten clean for five days, you get to enjoy two treat meals on Saturday and Sunday. Long-term success will come only from enjoying two treat meals. Remember, your brain hates deprivation and needs to feel like there is a light at the end of the tunnel—a bright light! Basically, you'll replace two of your weekend meals with treat meals. This is the only meal plan that allows for this. I call this "tricking the brain" into feeling satisfied and ready to return to your good foods! Examples of treat meals include:

* Dinner with friends, in which you eat what you want including drinks and dessert (1,200–1,500 calories)

* Candy (5-ounce package of peanut M&M's) and medium popcorn at the movies (1,100 calories)

* A Sunday-morning brunch of eggs Benedict, ham, and tomatoes (780 calories)

I treat myself to all of these foods, guilt-free, knowing that on Monday I resume my five days of clean eating. Because I haven't said no to myself, I am happy and not deprived. Here are several guidelines and tips for managing your treat meals:

1. You can have your treat meals only if you've eaten completely clean for five days in a row. Having treat meals won't work otherwise.

2. *Treat meal* doesn't mean a full-day free-for-all. Your treat meals shouldn't be more than fifteen hundred calories each or you will regain hard-lost pounds. That still gives you a lot of leeway with what you can have.

3. Immediately throw leftover treat meals away. They will only cause you to eat more of a bad thing or indulge on a clean day.

4. Plan your treat meals. If you're going to dinner at a restaurant, for example, eat your clean meals at breakfast and lunch, then indulge in your treat meal at dinner.

With treat meals, you have structure and flexibility with a way to get thin that feels good. This is the only way of eating that works in my life and those of countless other people. This is a lifestyle and not a diet. What is amazing about eating clean for five days is that you break your addiction to sugar and kill cravings. I call this my "work hard, play hard" principle applied to food. Work hard and eat to live during the week, then play hard and live to eat for your treat meals.

An Overview of My 5 + 2 Eating Plan

* Begin my 5 + 2 Plan only after you've completed the two-week jump start.

* Each day, eat five meals: breakfast, lunch, and dinner, plus a midmorning and midafternoon snack.

* Choose four proteins, three vegetables, two fruits, two grains, and one fat from the hormone balancer/detox list of foods.

* Eat a serving of protein at breakfast, lunch, dinner, and one snack. Add a slow-digesting carb, such as a vegetable, oatmeal, beans or legumes, whole-grain bread, or brown rice, at lunch and dinner.

* Limit your intake of whole grains to no more than twice a day. An example would be your morning oatmeal and then a slice of whole-grain bread with lunch or dinner. Another example would be whole-grain toast in the morning and brown rice at dinner.

* Add veggies to two of your meals and one snack or to a whey protein shake.

* Eat one snack or meal daily with a clean fat, such as avocado, nuts or seeds, or flaxseed oil.

* Eat low-fat dairy foods (including hard cheeses) sparingly—no more than two servings a day. But remember: no milk.

* Eat two servings of fresh fruit daily. Enjoy them with meals, as desserts, or as snacks, and try to combine them with some protein.

SHAKE IN YOUR NUTRIENTS!

I HAVE A COUPLE of great tricks I use every day to sneak in my assigned nutrients. First, I blend a whey protein shake every morning adding the following: 1 handful of fresh or frozen spinach (the fruit cuts its strong green flavor), 1 cup of frozen mixed berries, the recommended daily dose of flaxseed oil, amino acid powder, water, and ice. This is packed with three of your allotted foods before you even start your day. I drink it every day! To get the rest of daily veggies in, simply have a salad for lunch and grilled veggies for dinner. Get a low-sugar whey isolate protein powder from any vitamin shop or drugstore.

Second, I microwave frozen broccoli (a cup) and gulp it down like a vitamin. Start thinking of veggies as easy-to-eat fat burners. Eat a protein, such as beans, on your lunch salad. For dinner, have fish or chicken with your veggies.

* Eat a variety of foods each week. Rotate your fruits, veggies, and protein selections frequently.

* Drink three liters of water daily.

* Enjoy two treat meals on the weekend.

Keep a Food Journal

Writing down what you eat each day practically guarantees greater weight loss. According to researchers at Kaiser Permanente's Center for Health Research, keeping a record of what you eat encourages you to take in fewer calories by forcing you to reflect on how much you're eating. The researchers found that dieters who wrote down what they ate for six months lost about thirteen pounds—double the amount of those who didn't journal their daily diet.

As you lose pounds, you'll gain something else: a greater understanding of why and when you overeat. You may learn that you overeat when you're stressed, that you snack at night, or that you're skipping meals. Your food journal forces you to be accountable for what you're putting into your body. It also can clue you into food patterns that keep you from reaching your weight goal.

Starting and maintaining a good food journal is simple and takes just a few minutes a day. I've provided a sample food journal for you in appendix B. Write down exactly what you eat every day, including quantities. Put a smiley face next to clean-eating days and make positive notes to yourself when you have a successful day. If you eat something you didn't plan to eat, write that down, too. Fill out everything as completely as you can. Be accurate and be honest, because you're not fooling anyone but yourself.

At the end of each week, scrutinize the information you've recorded in your journal. Chances are, you'll notice some patterns. Spotting those patterns and learning ways to overcome them will lead to long-lasting weight loss. When you first start keeping track, it can feel tedious. It will get easier as it becomes a fun, healthy routine.

Foods to Avoid: Hormone Imbalancers and Toxic Foods

Unless eaten as part of your treat meals, there are foods that you should avoid. These include fast-digesting carbs such as white breads, bagels, potatoes, and white rice, and sweets like honey, jams, jellies, syrups, table sugar, candies, soft drinks, fruit juice, cakes, and pies. Fast-digesting carbs break down fast and trigger hormonal imbalances (think insulin) that cause you to store more of what you eat as fat. Other hormone imbalancers and toxic foods include milk, processed and cured meats, and any foods containing trans fats. Here is a detailed list of what to avoid:

Proteins

Bacon

Sausage

Fried fish, poultry, and meats

Fatty meats

Processed meats

Milk

Cream

Regular yogurt

Ice cream or ice milk

Carbohydrates

Bagels

Cakes

Candy, sweets, desserts

Cookies

Cornflakes

Corn pasta

Couscous

Cream of wheat, instant

French baguette bread

French fries

Hamburger, hot dog rolls

Italian white bread

Long-grain white rice

Middle Eastern flatbread

Pies

White potatoes

Processed, packaged cereals

Refined sugar, high-fructose corn syrup, sugar alcohols (mannitol, maltitol, sorbitol), and artificial sweeteners (aspartame, NutraSweet, Splenda)

Rice Chex

Sugar jellies, jams, or preserves

Syrups

White rice

Udon Japanese noodles

Fats

Bacon fat

Butter

Creamy full-fat salad dressings or
   mayonnaise

Lard

Shortening

Trans fats, including margarine

Beverages

Blended coffee drinks

Juice

Mixed alcoholic beverages
   and cocktails

Punches

Sodas, including diet sodas

Yogurt drinks

Calories Count

Let me be clear about calories: You will gain weight when you eat more calories than your metabolism can burn off. A calorie overload triggers hormone reactions that turn those excess calories into fat and pack it directly on your belly, hips, butt, and thighs. It takes around thirty-five hundred calories to add one pound of fat to your body. If you want to lose weight, you'd better be in a calorie deficit. In other words, eat fewer calories each day than you burn off.

In order to lose one pound a week, you need to create a weekly caloric deficit of thirty-five hundred calories, or five hundred fewer calories a day (500 x 7 days = 1 pound of weight loss per week). This means that by cutting out five hundred calories of unnecessary calories each day, or burning five hundred calories a day by exercising—or both—you'd be able to drop a pound or more a week. On average, you can eat fifteen to eighteen hundred calories a day to lose around two pounds a week, as long as you stay active.

During your five days of clean eating, however, you don't have to count calories. I have done that for you. If you choose your foods correctly, you'll already be eating the right amount of calories to burn fat. I do recommend, however, that you make sure your treat meals are never over fifteen hundred calories. You can read labels or go online to check popular junk and restaurant foods. You already know that restaurant-size pasta is just under your fifteen-hundred-calorie mark. You don't want to eat in excess of three thousand total calories on the days you enjoy treat meals.

SMALL CALORIE CUTS MAKE A BIG DIFFERENCE

GIVE UP THIS . . .	LOSE THIS MUCH WEIGHT IN A MONTH . . .
3 soft drinks a day	4 pounds
1 large bagel a day	3 pounds
1 large bowl of chocolate ice cream nightly	4 pounds
Snacking on 15 to 20 potato chips a day	2 pounds
3 fast-food value meals a week	4 pounds
2 nightly glasses of wine	2 pounds

Alcohol Makes You Chubby

I can always tell when new clients drink too frequently. They have that soft, doughy appearance. If you're really serious about losing weight and getting lean, you have to rethink your drinking habits. Alcohol causes your body to pump out more estrogen and less testosterone. Over time, this hormonal imbalance will make you fat. Excessive consumption of alcohol strains your liver, which responds by slowing down on fat burning. Alcohol also dehydrates your body, and this only adds bloat to your face. Not to mention the calorie count: A five-ounce glass of wine has 120 calories, so even a little drinking can throw off your diet in a big way. Plus, wine is higher in fast-digesting carbs than clear liquors such as vodka, so it tends to pack on weight more easily.

The worst of the worst are mixed drinks like margaritas or piña coladas, as well as juice-based drinks. Some of these drinks have as many calories in them (or more) as a slice of cheesecake (four hundred calories). Spend a few hours at a bar on Friday night, drinking some of these, and you could easily consume three thousand calories in drinks! And if you're anything like me, drinking leads to major food cravings. I cut my drinking down severely because alcohol always makes me overeat.

So ask yourself: Would you rather have one mixed drink or a slice of cheesecake? I would go for the cheesecake every time. Honestly, mixed drinks should never touch your lips again, unless as part of a treat meal. They are a total waste of calories. I drink only vodka and soda or tequila over ice to avoid all those empty calories. Here is a list of calorie counts for alcoholic beverages, from good to bad, so you can see what they will cost you.

CALORIES IN ALCOHOLIC DRINKS

DRINK	SERVING SIZE	CALORIES
Tequila, 80 proof	1.4 fluid oz.	97
Champagne	5 oz.	98
Bourbon, 80 proof	1.4 fluid oz.	100
Vodka, 80 proof	1.4 fluid oz.	103
Scotch, 80 proof	1.4 fluid oz.	103
Beer, light	12 fluid oz.	103
White wine, dry	5 fluid oz.	120
Bloody Mary	10 fluid oz.	125
Red wine (Cabernet, Merlot)	5 fluid oz.	129
Martini, vodka or gin	Regular martini glass	135
Gin and tonic	6 fluid oz.	143
Beer, regular	12 fluid oz.	145
Sex on the Beach	Standard cocktail glass	150
Screwdriver	Standard cocktail glass	180
Dirty vodka martini	Regular martini glass	210
Cosmopolitan	Regular martini glass	213
Mai tai	Standard cocktail glass	225
Appletini	Regular martini glass	235
Vodka soda (bottled)	12 fluid oz.	253
Long Island iced tea	8 fluid oz.	276
Mojito	8 fluid oz.	325
Margarita, frozen	8 fluid oz.	376
Piña colada	8 fluid oz.	443
Daiquiri	8 fluid oz.	449

Here's how to handle the alcohol issue: Stick to my eat-clean plan for five days—that means no alcohol—and if you want to enjoy a drink, make it part of your treat meal, or cut back drastically. If you have cocktails every night after work, for example, go from two drinks to one. And if you like mixed drinks, have them made with club soda or water to save on calories. You can lose up to a pound a week just by cutting your alcohol intake in half.

> ## LOSE THE LIQUID CALORIES!
>
> **LIQUID CALORIES IN** alcohol, juices, or sodas are sneaky; their impact on your weight can be enormous. Scientific evidence confirms that the calories in these liquids don't suppress your hunger like the calories in certain solid foods do.
>
> Since liquid calories don't make you feel full, cutting back on them shouldn't make you feel deprived.
>
> Lose the juice! It's nothing but liquid sugar. Most of the fat-fighting fiber in fruit is lost when it's turned into juice. For example, an orange contains about three grams of fiber. It takes about six cups of orange juice to reach the three grams of fiber in an orange. Plus, when produce is turned into juice or puree, it loses nutrients like potassium and vitamin C.

Variety, Variety, Variety

Like every teenager, I was obsessed with losing weight. I remember taking Nutrition 101 during my first year of college, and I asked my teacher, "How do you lose weight?" She paused to think for a moment and then said, "Variety, variety, variety." What she meant by this is that eating many different foods ensures that you get a number of fat-burning nutrients and prevents boredom (and therefore bingeing). Remember, weight loss is a mind game, and boredom leads to cheating. I recommend that you try a new food each week, and to boost nutrition, stick with foods in their most natural form.

The secret, then, to getting hot and healthy is to eat clean foods that balance your hormones, detox your body, and burn fat for five days in a row, then plan your treat meals carefully and enjoy! Doesn't this sound like a more fun, interesting way to lose weight? With my plan, you can have it all.

6 Get Thin in the Real World

A lot of diet books have rigid, hard-to-follow plans that are impractical for most people's lifestyles. Success comes from knowing how and what to eat no matter where you are—which is why I'm all about showing you how to eat clean in the real world. But here's what you're up against: The food industry cuts corners, adds toxins, and has no interest in your health. The more processed a food is, the more profitable it is, and processing typically makes foods less healthy. If the food industry really cared about promoting healthier eating, apples and bananas, instead of cookies and chip bags, would be used as enticers at supermarket checkout aisles. But healthy, clean foods like fresh fruits and vegetables obviously aren't where food companies look for profits. Producing clean foods isn't a big moneymaker! Even so, you can get thin in the real world, as long as you have the information to make the right choices.

You're a Rat in a Maze of Food

The ever-present food marketing, especially from companies pushing unhealthy products, is impossible to get away from and seems to be literally shoved down your throat. You are a rat in a food maze at the grocery store, in front of your television, and just in your every-day route to and from work. Your mind is constantly being stimulated by packaging and commercials that make you hungry—but not for the good stuff. No, you crave the cheap, calorie-loaded, chemically enhanced junk food. That's consumerism, folks.

The food industry will also do everything it can to minimize health concerns associated with its products, like airing commercials designed to get you to eat unhealthy junk. My favorite commercial was funded by an organization to promote good feelings about high-fructose corn syrup. I laugh out loud every time I see it. Then I get furious because I know that these marketers know they are poisoning America for profit. This is evil, and this is the industry entrusted to feed us!

Go Organic

One of the greatest ways you can eat clean and lose weight is to stock up on organic foods. When you buy organic, you:

* Avoid artificial ingredients. This includes synthetic colors and flavors.

* Cut bad fats from your diet. Trans fats are not allowed in organic food. Irradiated or genetically engineered ingredients also don't make the cut.

* Limit your exposure to pesticides. By law, organic produce can't be treated with synthetic pesticides. Hormones, steroids, and antibiotics are also banned from organic meat, dairy, and poultry.

* Protect the environment. Organic farming reduces water contamination, improves soil quality, and protects wildlife habitats.

THE FOOD INDUSTRY laces foods with additives, preservatives, and colorings to make them taste better and last longer on the shelves. Unfortunately, these foods are making us fatter and unhealthier by the day! I want to keep you from eating the chemicals put in your food by the food industry—chemicals that are making you fat and sick. With fewer chemicals messing up your system, your body can regulate fat loss more efficiently. You'll start feeling better and looking thinner as a result. Here's a look at some of the most dangerous additives and the foods and products they're in.

ADDITIVE	DANGERS	FOODS AND PRODUCTS WITH THIS ADDITIVE
Artificial coloring	Immune system damage, accelerated aging, increased risk of cancer	Cherries in fruit cocktail Canned juices Cereals Sausage Candy Gelatin Commercially baked goods Skin of some Florida oranges (citrus red 2) Soft drinks
Nitrate	Increased risk of cancer	Hot dogs Bacon Ham Processed meats
Paraben	Mimics estrogen in the body—which makes you fat; paraben has been found in breast cancer tumors	Soap Toothpaste Hair-care products Lotions Processed vegetables Salad dressings Natural vanilla extract Jelly coatings of meat products Dried meat products Cereal- or potato-based snacks Coated nuts Candy (excluding chocolate)

ADDITIVE	DANGERS	FOODS AND PRODUCTS WITH THIS ADDITIVE
Sodium benzoate, benzoic acid	Increased risk of cancer, including leukemia	Soft drinks Diet soft drinks Noncarbonated soft drinks Fruit juices Pickles Beer
MSG (monosodium glutamate)	Stimulates the appetite; an unnecessary source of salt in the diet; can cause allergic reactions	Soups Salad dressings Chips Frozen non-organic entrées Frozen meats Restaurant foods

On top of all that, organic food tastes better, stays fresher longer, and tends to have higher levels of nutrients than conventional foods. Look for the USDA stamp certifying that food is organic.

If your grocery store doesn't carry enough organic food for your liking, ask for a manager and demand more organic products. The store will listen and document your request. Remember, it's all about money. If a store sees the demand, it will ask its buyers to meet it. You can be part of a wonderful movement that will enrich your community.

> *Quick Tip:* You can lose weight fast by eating frozen, pre-packaged meals—as long as they're from an organic market. These foods are generally sugar- and calorie-controlled and make calorie counting a breeze. Buying healthy pre-packaged meals is convenient, too—perfect for lunch or dinner, or to take to work.

Label Reading Made Easy

People always ask me whether they should read labels and worry about carbs and fat content. Answer: No! You don't need to overcomplicate your grocery shopping trip by trying to decipher everything on a food label.

I've got a simple rule. Pay attention to three things only:

* *The amount of sugar.* Total sugar is listed in grams, and your goal is to not exceed five to nine grams per serving. Your body doesn't even register less than five grams, which means no insulin spikes and no fat storing. Eating a full meal under five grams is difficult to do, however, so I recommend eating no more than nine grams. All of my meals are prepared with that in mind. You will notice that most foods low in sugar and calories are also low in the other bad things, like saturated fats.

* *The number of calories per serving.* Based on a 1,500-calorie-a-day diet, make sure a product has no more than 150 calories per *snack* serving or 450 calories per *meal* serving and is under nine grams of sugar. (Men can eat 500 calories per meal and 150 calories per snack to start.)

* *The serving size.* Don't be fooled by serving size. Some packages are not single servings; they contain multiple servings. I buy only meals that have the right calories per container. Why? I don't have the willpower to *not* eat the whole container in one sitting. If you don't think you can eat one serving of enchilada when there are two in the container, don't buy it!

Low-Fat Versus Nonfat

Did we learn nothing from the fat-free craze? I was in my twenties when it hit, and tons of delicious desserts were being pushed as healthy. I stocked my fridge full of fat-free coffee cakes, raspberry tarts, and cookies. It seemed too good to be true, and it was. Close to a hundred million of us are overweight or obese, according to the National Institutes of Health, a 50 percent increase since the 1970s fat-free products first hit the market.

What I can't understand is how many still believe in this fat-free lie. Most nonfat products are pumped full of fast-digesting carbs to replace the fat: potato starch, cornstarch, dextrins (a simple sugar), maltodextrins, polydextrose (another simple sugar), and gums, to name just a few. So if you're chowing down on fat-free foods, you're ingesting loads of sugar. And sugar makes you fat, as I love to remind everyone! I actually suggest to my clients that they choose low-fat foods instead of nonfat foods in order to avoid the sugar. *Low-fat* technically means that the product has three grams of fat or less per serving. But it also means that some of the fat has merely been removed, rather than fully replaced with sugary, fat-forming carbs. So if you have a choice, opt for low-fat over fat-free.

Low-Calorie

You might think you're making a good food choice when you eat a product labeled "low-cal," but in reality you're often being tricked into buying some nasty additives and artificial sweeteners. Artificial sweeteners can trick your body into gaining weight and are dangerous to your health. When my brother was in high school, he worked behind the counter of a movie snack stand. He told me that the metal tubings used to dispense diet soda eroded so quickly that they had to be replaced monthly. What do you think that same sweetener is doing to your insides? That made me cut back!

According to research from the University of Texas Health Science Center at San Antonio, the more diet soda people drank on a daily basis, the greater risk they had of becoming overweight. The researchers believe that the artificial sweeteners in diet drinks actually increase food cravings. If you must use artificial sweeteners and don't have access to Truvia (a stevia-based product), one to two packets a day are the most you should consume. But try to do without if possible.

No Sugar Added

If you see a food or coffee drink marketed as "no sugar added," run the other way, because it's anything but. This is the most deceptive packaging of all. Foods that make this claim are usually sweetened with apple or white grape juice concentrate, which is no different from white sugar. It's so fattening! Or the so-called sugar-free food may be laced with sugar alcohols (see the box), which do contain calories. "No sugar added" is yet another lie the food industry uses to entice you.

THE SUGAR-FREE SCOOP: SUGAR ALCOHOLS

Many foods (including protein bars) and beverages are sweetened with substances called sugar alcohols (such as sorbitol, lactitol, mannitol, maltitol, and xylitol). Sugar alcohol is formed by combining an acid with a sugar, and is nothing more than a carb. Foods containing them are labeled "sugar-free," but they are not calorie-free. They provide about half the calories of sugar and can still make you gain weight, so you don't want to go overboard. The other big downside to sugar alcohols is that they can cause gastrointestinal cramps, bloating, loose stools, and diarrhea.

Grocery Shopping for Weight Loss

Okay, now you know how to decode labels and you see the differences among food products. So let's go grocery shopping. One of my favorite things to do with clients is take them on a grocery trip. It's so important for them to show me what they like to eat, and then I can make small changes or guide them in a smarter direction. I want people to understand that there are many tasty, healthy options out there—and also to know that many of the foods they think are good for them are causing weight gain and depression.

So go with me to the grocery store. To avoid pricey impulse purchases, make a shopping list first, and don't go to the store hungry or with your kids.

Okay, grab a cart. Here's how to load your cabinets, refrigerator, and freezer with the best choices your grocery store has to offer. After you return home to unload, you'll be just that much closer to getting thin.

The Produce Section

First, we're going to shop the outer perimeter. That's where the really clean, healthy stuff is (as opposed to the middle of the store, where all the boxed, processed stuff is lying in wait). Begin with the produce section. My tips:

* Choose mostly raw, fresh, and preferably organic vegetables.

* When purchasing a salad mix, look for the most colorful greens in the bag. The more color, the more healthful antioxidants in the salad.

* Berries are very perishable. At the store, check for freshness by looking at the bottom of the package. If you see a stain, this means the fruit has been bruised or is overripe. It will spoil fast.

The Dairy Section

* Next, pick up dairy products, such as low-fat cottage cheese and other low-fat cheeses, and Greek-style yogurt. Be sure to choose the additive-free versions.

* Stay away from soft, pasteurized, or artificially colored cheese products. They're high in saturated fat, dyes, and preservatives.

* Choose organic free-range eggs if available. Organic eggs are free of the toxic hormones and antibiotics pumped into factory-produced eggs.

The Fish Counter

Many varieties of fish are loaded with fat-burning omega-3 fatty acids. The types with the most omega-3s include the rich, oily, dark-fleshed fish, such as salmon, sardines, bluefin tuna, and trout. Also, choose any freshwater white fish, and steer clear of seafood that has been breaded or fried. Canned light meat tuna (water-packed) is fine, too; you'll find that in the canned-meat aisle.

The Poultry and Meat Department

Work your way over to the poultry and meat department for turkey, chicken, and meat.

* Select low-fat organic poultry such as chicken or turkey breasts. Avoid self-basting turkeys, which have fat injected into them. Eat lean ground turkey and chicken that contains less skin, which is very high in fat and calories.

* Choose organic meats, if possible. Factory-farmed meats (and poultry) contain hormones and antibiotics that upset your hormonal, immune, and digestive systems.

The Whole-Grain Aisles: Breads, Cereals, and Grains

Here, you'll want to opt for whole grains over refined products (such as white rice and white flour) so that you get more fiber, folic acid, magnesium, vitamins E and B_6, copper, zinc, and dozens of phytochemicals. Make sure you're getting whole grains (just because bread is brown doesn't make it whole grain). The product is whole grain if the first ingredient on the label is whole grain, whole wheat, or rye (plain wheat flour is not whole grain).

* Choose all whole grains and foods containing whole grains, including cereals, breads, whole-grain crackers, oatmeal, brown rice, and wild rice.

* Steer clear of all white flour products, white rice, and white pasta. White products generally contain additives and preservatives that you won't find in whole-grain foods.

The Beans/Legumes Aisle

Learn to love beans and legumes. These foods are vegetarian proteins with abundant nutrition, including lots of fiber. One-half cup of beans contains as much protein as three ounces of broiled steak or chicken breast. Canned and dried beans offer the same nutrition; just be sure to rinse canned beans to remove excess salt before using, or select no-salt-added products. Choose beans cooked without animal fat.

The Soup Aisle

Your best choices are salt- and fat-free bean, lentil, pea, vegetable, barley, and brown rice soups. Select organic products if available. Avoid canned soups made with preservatives, MSG, or fat as well as all creamed soups. There are lots of varieties of canned soups made without added chemicals.

The Frozen-Food Section

Frozen produce without added sugar, fat, or sauce is a good choice. Frozen fruits and vegetables are often as nutritious as (and sometimes more so than) their fresh counterparts since they're frozen immediately after harvest. The frozen vegetable blends make planning healthy meals easy. Frozen fruits are great for smoothies, as long as they contain no added sugar.

The Nuts and Seeds Aisle

Nuts and seeds are rich in monounsaturated fat, the same fat found in olive oil, which helps raise our good cholesterol (HDL) levels without raising our bad cholesterol (LDL) levels. Walnuts are especially rich in alpha-linolenic acid, which the body converts to fat-burning omega-3 fatty acids. Almonds are a great source of calcium.

* Go for all fresh, raw nuts.

* Avoid salted, oiled, or roasted nuts.

* Select nut butters, such as peanut butter or raw almond butter. Choose organic products, if possible.

The Oil Aisle

Here, you'll want to choose cold-pressed olive oil, flaxseed oil, and canola oil. Avoid all saturated fats, hydrogenated margarine, refined processed oils, shortenings, and hardened oils. Low-fat salad dressings and low-fat mayo are good choices, too.

The Seasonings Aisle

You're going to need some spices and condiments on hand to prepare the recipes in the appendix. For example:

Garlic powder

Onion powder

Dried herbs (such as basil and oregano)

Ground cumin

Vinegar (red wine and balsamic)

Dijon mustard

Ground cinnamon

Chicken or vegetable broth

Salsa

Eat Rich for Cheap

If you haven't been buying healthy, organic foods because you think they will break your budget, think again. Switching to a diet of mostly low-sugar, natural foods can shave up to six hundred dollars per year off your family's grocery bill, according to a study in the *Journal of the American Dietetic Association*. But you must buy healthy foods instead of, not in addition to, junk food. This means your shopping cart should be filled with whole-grain products and fruits and vegetables. Eating organic doesn't mean you have to break the bank. Here are some tips:

* Find a local farmer's market. Prices are typically lower.

* Eat organic produce and meat. You will lose all the added hormones that cause you to gain weight.

* Buying in-season organic can be cheaper than out-of-season conventional.

* Buy in bulk for items like grains, nuts, and beans.

Good, Bad, and Ugly—Eating Out at Restaurants

If you're like most people, you find yourself eating out at restaurants a lot: You get tired of cooking at home all the time, or you have work dinners. Fortunately, eating out doesn't have to mean pigging out, as long as you know how to make good choices. To help you do that, I've categorized restaurant foods into the "good, bad, and ugly." The trick is to choose mostly the good, ease off the bad, and don't order the ugly.

Mexican Restaurants

I love Mexican food, and there are lots of ways to enjoy it. I don't fill up on chips, and I never drink margaritas. Instead, I order chicken fajitas, and I eat the veggie and chicken filling first. Then, when I'm almost full, I enjoy a regular fajita wrapped in a flour tortilla.

Good

* Salsa. Not only is salsa fat-free, but it's also full of vitamins and phytochemicals. Load up your tacos, tortillas, or fajitas with salsa instead of sour cream and high-fat alternatives.

* Fajitas. Build them with chicken, vegetables, and salsa, rather than with high-fat items such as cheese and sour cream.

* Chicken soft tacos (420 calories).

* Shrimp tacos (490 calories).

* Any entrée with grilled chicken and rice.

Bad

* Quesadillas (900–1,400 calories).

* Taco salad with beef (1,450 calories).

Ugly

* Chicken burrito (1,530 calories).

* Stacked nachos (2,700 calories).

* Tortilla chips. Just fifteen of these triangles pack 192 calories.

Italian Restaurants

Good

* Protein entrées (such as fish, skinless chicken, or lean veal) with a side of vegetables rather than carbohydrate-rich pasta.

* Meatballs without the pasta, or served with spaghetti squash.

* Minestrone, a vegetable-rich soup that can help reduce your appetite for relatively few calories. Research shows that a soup starter can help curb your appetite—and your calorie intake.

* Red (tomato-based) sauce instead of white sauces, which are generally cream- and/or butter-based.

* Shellfish. Steamed or in a tomato-based broth, mussels, clams, and other shellfish are delicious, low-calorie choices.

Bad

* Garlic bread—two small slices (273 calories).

* Lasagna (1,000 calories).

Ugly

* Chicken Parmesan (1,300 calories). Chicken is lean, but not when it's fried and smothered in cheese!

* "Personal" deep-dish pizza (2,300 calories).

* Spaghetti and meatballs with meat sauce (2,430 calories).

Steak Houses

Good

* Filets and sirloins. They're the two leanest cuts of beef you can order.

* Barbecued chicken breast or a grilled fish entrée.

* House (mixed or green) salad with salad dressing on the side.

Bad

* New York strip, T-bone, porterhouse, or prime rib. You'll swallow tons of bad fat with these cuts.

* Caesar salad (this can cost you up to 900 calories).

Ugly

* An order of cheese fries with ranch dressing (3,000 calories).

Breakfast Restaurants

Good

* Two eggs, fruit salad, and an English muffin (470 calories).

* Scrambled egg whites or egg substitute (70–140 calories).

* Oatmeal with fruit salad—hold the butter and brown sugar (220 calories).

Bad

* Pancakes or waffles (900 calories).

Ugly

* French toast with syrup and sausage or bacon (1,300 calories).

* Stacked and stuffed hotcakes with syrup (1,500 calories).

Asian Restaurants

I love Asian food, too. Generally, I eat steamed dishes that have veggies and meat. Stay away from anything that's battered.

Good

* Steamed chicken and broccoli (280 calories).

* Shrimp with lobster sauce (400 calories).

* Tuna sashimi (240 calories).

* A cup of miso, egg drop, or hot-and-sour soup (40–100 calories).

* Steamed Asian vegetables—baby corn, snap peas, water chestnuts, and sprouts (200 calories).

Bad

* Egg rolls (190 calories).

Ugly

* Tempura rolls (544 calories). The word *tempura* is code for "battered and deep-fried."

* A bowl of wonton soup (690 calories).

* General Tso's chicken (1,300 calories).

* Sweet-and-sour pork (1,300 calories).

* Lemon chicken (1,400 calories).

* Fried rice (1,500 calories).

* Kung Pao chicken (1,620 calories).

* Pork lo mein (1,820 calories).

Fast-Food Restaurants

Good

* Veggie burger (330 calories).

* Grilled chicken sandwiches (360–570 calories).

* Entrée salads with dressing (310–500 calories).

Bad

* Bacon cheeseburger (580 calories).

* King-size order of fries (600 calories).

Ugly

* Big Mac Value Meal (1,170 calories).

* Triple burger with cheese (970 calories).

* Whopper with cheese (1,100 calories).

* Value Meals (1,300–2,100 calories).

COFFEE DRINKS ARE sabotaging your weight loss! Some of them contain calories equivalent to a piece of chocolate cake. That sucks! I'd rather eat the cake than drink my calories. Use coffee for what it is: a way to wake up and feel human in the morning. You should never exceed two cups a day anyway. Ask for regular coffee and add your own low-fat milk and sweetener. Be careful: Some coffeehouses offer drinks with "no sugar added." They are deceptive because the products still have sugar in them. Here's a look at the calorie counts in some common coffee drinks, along with some smarter alternatives.

COFFEE DRINKS	ALTERNATIVES
Vanilla latte made with whole milk, 16 oz.: 320 calories	Fat-free latte, 16 oz.: 100 calories
Cappuccino made with whole milk, 12 oz.: 150 calories	Cappuccino made with nonfat milk, 12 oz.: 100 calories
White chocolate mocha made with whole milk, 12 oz.: 510 calories	Coffee with nonfat milk, 12 oz.: 50 calories
Frappuccino, 16 oz.: 470–560 calories	Frappuccino lite, 16 oz.: 150 calories
Iced chocolate mocha: 534 calories	Coffee, regular or decaf, 12 oz.: 10 calories

7 Ways to Not Break the Plan When Eating Out

1. Call ahead or visit the restaurant's Web site before you eat out. Many restaurant chains, such as Applebee's, Ruby Tuesday, Chili's, and Olive Garden, publish their nutritional information. If you look at the menu but can't resist what's on it, don't go!

2. Decide what you'll order before you go. This helps you stay on track and decreases temptation.

3. Ask the waiter to hold the bread, or at least move it to the side of the table (away from you!).

4. When you're eating out on clean days, order meat entrées, veggie dishes, and salad.

5. Order sauces and dressings on the side. Share entrées with a companion or save one-half of your entrée for another meal. I ask for a doggie bag at the beginning of my meal and fill it with any food on my plate that exceeds one portion size.

6. Be assertive. Ask about preparation methods so you can make better choices. Ask if soups are made with flour; if they are, don't order them. Avoid foods that are fried, sautéed, or cooked in heavy cream sauces.

7. Practice portion control. One protein serving is about the size of the palm of your hand. One serving of rice, pasta, or mashed potatoes is about as big as your fist.

NOT SO FAST!

FAST-FOOD RESTAURANTS can be deceptive in their nutritional information, too, so watch out. Subway has its "seven sandwiches with six grams of fat or less" category; nutritional information includes almost all of the available vegetable toppings, which are naturally low in calories and high in nutrients. But adding ingredients like mayo, ranch dressing, oils, and cheese (which almost everyone orders) increases calorie and fat content greatly. In fact, a six-inch veggie sandwich with two slices of cheddar cheese and one tablespoon of regular mayonnaise contains four hundred calories and twenty grams of fat. The massive quantity of bread alone makes it a poor restaurant choice. Although Subway has healthier selections than most fast-food joints and prints a listing of additives, the catchy "Seven Under Six" slogan demonstrates the misuse of statistics for advertising purposes.

The sandwiches are only low-fat or low-cal if you get lean meat, without the mayo, oil, cheese, dressing, or sauces. That means ordering basically a turkey on whole wheat with veggies and mustard only—haha. I always remove half the bun or get a spinach salad with low-fat ranch dressing and chicken. No matter where you eat today, exercise healthy skepticism. Evaluate nutritional information available in the restaurant.

How to Stay with It

I've noticed that most diet lapses come after about ninety days. However, they are avoidable. Here are some tips to help you stay on track:

* *Clean house.* Remove *all* junk from your kitchen. If you were a heroin addict, would you keep smack in the house? How can you possibly resist cravings if your favorite junk food is three feet away? Clear your kitchen of trigger foods like ice cream, potato chips, candy, and any highly addictive junk food, so that if you have the desire to go on a binge, you'd have to drive to the store for whatever you're craving. You are less likely to cheat if you have to get out of your pajamas, into your car, and drive somewhere for your junk food.

* *Be choosy about your dishes.* As the size of your plate or bowl increases, so will the amount of food you dish out and eat. An experiment conducted by researchers at the University of Illinois at Urbana-Champaign confirmed just that: Of the eighty-five participants, those who were given thirty-four-ounce bowls scooped out a third more ice cream than those given seventeen-ounce bowls. If you're eating at home, serve dinner on large salad plates (seven to nine inches in diameter) instead of traditional twelve-inch dinner plates. Always put food on dishes! Eating straight from a box, bag, or serving bowl is a recipe for regret.

* *Don't eat in front of the television.* The more time you spend in front of the TV, the more likely you are to gain weight. Worst of all is watching your favorite show: When you're really distracted, you can completely lose track of how much food you've put in your mouth.

* *Enlist support.* Trying to lose weight can feel like a lonely uphill battle. It becomes so important to have a support team. Rather than feeling like it's you against the world, you can get your friends and loved ones involved in your cause. Arm yourself with a few simple replies, such as, "You're right, one cookie won't hurt me, but it won't help me lose weight, either." Also, explain what you need in terms of support in a way that doesn't put the other person on the defensive, such as, "I appreciate that you brought home dinner, but I need you

to respect my desire to get in shape and not surprise me with fattening food." Basically, you'll want to point out behaviors that drive you to cheat and ask for everyone's support. If you stick to your guns, you'll build support and respect. People will look to you for answers about nutrition and weight loss. The student becomes the teacher, and you will start inspiring those around you.

* ***Keep lists.*** Write down a list of reasons why you don't want to be fat, like "I will have to wear fat clothes, and I won't feel attractive"; as well as a list of things you love about being thin, like "I'll feel in control of my life," or "I will feel strong and sexy." Keep your list in front of you at all times. Also, post a before picture or picture of you that isn't flattering on your fridge or desktop as a reminder of why you want to stay on track.

Staying thin and healthy for life depends on making easy changes you can sustain for as long as you live. You will succeed with this plan because you won't feel deprived and you will have so much more energy for living. But diet is only part of the picture. Next, I'm going to show you how to exercise with a workout program that requires very little time, but produces wonderful results.

Part 3

THIS IS HOW YOU EXERCISE TO GET HOT AND HEALTHY

7 20 Minutes to a Faster Metabolism

My 2-Week Cardio Plan

When working with clients, I always try to balance my tough-love approach with happy news. And some of the happiest news I deliver is this: You can cut your cardio down to only twenty minutes.

With your workouts, it's not how long, but how strong. You can actually expend more calories in less time by doing shorter, harder cardio workouts. You'll not only burn calories but also boost your metabolic rate, so your body continues burning extra calories for up to several hours after your workout is over. Twenty minutes is all you need to make this happen.

Here's more good news: For the next two weeks, twenty minutes is the maximum time you need to spend on cardio—no resistance training yet, just cardio performed only five times a week. Within those twenty minutes, you'll do short bursts at full effort. This is called interval intensity training. The goal is to prep your body for fat burning by recharging your metabolism and boosting your calorie burn.

In This Chapter:

* *Burn more fat in less time*
* *How aerobic exercise burns fat and improves your mood*
* *Aerobic exercise and hormonal balance*
* *Using cardio machines more effectively*
* *Tips to increase calorie burn*

In these two weeks, you'll notice a loss of weight, better muscle tone (and higher metabolism), and more energy. Just because it's short, don't think this program is going to be easy. Interval intensity training makes you sweat your butt off, literally.

I believe that everyone has at least twenty minutes they can devote to themselves most days of the week. In fact, not only does twenty minutes make sense if you're crunched for time, but current research shows it's plenty of time to burn fat, especially if you exercise in intervals with intensity.

Also, this program works effectively if you're very out of shape or if you're in decent shape but want to take your workouts to a higher level. So start getting excited about this new two-week routine. There's really no excuse not to do it!

FAT-BURNING FACT: TRIPLE YOUR FAT LOSS WITH INTERVALS

YOU CAN TRIPLE your fat loss and shed pounds a lot faster with twenty-minute workouts that incorporate intervals. A study from the University of New South Wales in Australia shows just how fast: Researchers looked at forty-five lean and overweight women who cycled three times per week for fifteen weeks. Those who switched between sprinting on the bike for eight seconds and light pedaling for twelve seconds over a twenty-minute workout lost three times as much fat as the women who exercised at a moderate pace for a full forty minutes. And that's not all. Without even changing their diets, the sprinters also dropped five and a half pounds, on average, while the nonsprinters gained a pound.

Source: International Journal of Obesity

Cardio Power

My two-week cardio program uses the fat-burning muscle groups of the body: glutes (butt), hamstrings, and quadriceps. Typical cardio exercises include: walking, jogging, running, indoor cycling, swimming, or using cardio machines.

Cardio activity is important for several reasons. First, it's a fat burner. Aerobic exercise burns fat by increasing your body's fat-burning enzymes. These enzymes help your body burn more calories at rest. Aerobic exercise also improves oxygen delivery. More oxygen can get to your muscles, where it breaks down carbohydrates and fat into the fuel your body needs to move. When oxygen is present, more fat is burned.

Second, aerobic exercise strengthens your heart and lungs. Your heart pumps more blood with less effort and delivers more oxygen more efficiently. Your lung capacity is increased, allowing you to breathe in more oxygen. When you work out aerobically on a regular basis, any sluggish or out-of-breath feelings from exercise will eventually disappear. Putting the right amount of good stress on your heart and lungs through cardio exercises is imperative to keeping these organs strong and healthy.

Third, aerobic exercise has almost magical effects on your hormonal balance. It increases growth hormone, for example, and this really stimulates fat burning. Exercise moves glucose into muscle cells. This means your body doesn't have to use as much insulin. Less insulin decreases your chances of getting fat. Exercise also rebalances estrogen production, and increases progesterone levels.

Testosterone is affected, too. Workouts break down muscle protein. Your body responds by secreting more testosterone. Testosterone helps repair and rebuild muscle. The more muscle you have, the faster your metabolism.

In addition, exercise flushes out stress hormones from your body and elevates levels of feel-good endorphins. Endorphins are emotional tranquilizers that reduce stress and anxiety. When these brain chemicals are turned on consistently and in high doses, they addict you to working out. After a proper workout, you should feel a high that lasts throughout your day and affects all your personal connections with people. I am walking proof of someone who needs an endorphin high and relies on it to get through life. Exercise is a powerful cure to a sometimes sick and stressful environment. Do it right and you'll learn to crave exercise as much as you used to crave junk food. So along with diet, exercise is ideal for keeping your hormones and chemistry in balance.

My Aerobics Secrets

Let me define for you what my kind of workout means: exercising with intensity and consistency. Intensity is pushing yourself hard for shorter periods of time. The greater the intensity, the greater the fat burn.

Have you ever noticed the same women at the gym on those cardio machines for hours, yet they never lose a pound? That's because their bodies are no longer responding to the same old movement. What they're doing—long, slow cardio—is the least effective and most boring way to burn calories. They're not working out with enough intensity.

Most people just press the buttons on a piece of cardio equipment and do the time. If I see one more person doing their cardio while reading a magazine, I'll scream! That's a waste of time and does nothing for your body. Remember, it's not how long, but how strong you work out that counts.

I realize that some of you haven't ever really pushed yourself with cardio. There are many reasons for this. One big reason is that you probably associate the burning feeling of exercise with pain, sweat, and manual labor. It's tough to put yourself through those things voluntarily. To get over this and work out with greater intensity, you've got to break that association. Love the burn and love the sweat; don't run from them! Start equating them with results. They mean you're sculpting a sleek, slender body. Your body is changing for the better.

One more thing while I'm on the subject: You measure intensity by the burn and the sweat, too—not by heart rate. Unless you have heart problems, take off that heart monitor and ignore everything you've learned about staying in the heart rate range of 65 to 85 percent of your maximum heart rate. The more your muscles burn and the more you are drenched in sweat, the more intense your workout—and the more fat you're burning.

What also counts is consistency—sticking with it. If you slack off, you won't get results. The enemy of consistency is boredom. Let's face it: Most people dread cardio work if they think they have to hop on a machine for an hour after work. After a while, they'll start hating it, and they'll stop doing it. That's just human nature. My twenty-minute cardio program is definitely not boring. You'll be doing short cardio stints in which you're constantly changing things up.

Another reason people aren't consistent is that they don't see results fast enough. That won't happen here. After years of putting my clients on this program, I've been able to change their bodies in one week. That gets them hooked and excited about their future weight loss and tone. Not only do they drop weight, they also stick with the program. The same thing will happen to you.

Build a Better Body in 2 Weeks: My 20-Minute Programs

To burn fat and speed up your metabolism, put maximum effort into your workout and stick with it. Each of the following programs is progressive and uses intervals, which are key to fat burning. You'll start at a certain level of intensity, and I'll show you how to increase it. You'll be amazed by the progress you make each day you work out like this. These programs train your body to go longer at higher levels of effort and work at a higher percentage of your aerobic capacity. That burns more calories, helps you lose weight, and improves your overall health. Most importantly, you are prepping your body for the resistance routine to come.

You'll do five 20-minute cardio workouts each week. Follow my guidelines for each example. Remember: The harder and faster you go, the more fat you'll burn.

As for which machine or program to follow, the best one for you is the one that you like and are most apt to use. You've got to enjoy your activity. Choose one of the following machines and stick with only that machine for the two-week cardio prep. After that time, you can use different machines, but be sure to keep it intense.

The Treadmill Program

Treadmills can be found in most gyms, or you can buy a used one at a reasonable price for home use if you want your own. Make sure to buy a brand that will go to a 15 percent incline. The treadmill is a terrific cardio tool for getting rid of unwanted body fat, improving your overall health, and strengthening your legs. Walking on an incline is great for toning your thighs, butt, core, and back, as well as for increasing metabolism. For maximum fat burning, don't touch the supports, pump your arms, and always have your chest out, shoulders back, and eyes forward.

Also, always keep your body tight and pretend that you are made of steel like the Terminator. Never loosen your joints or slap down your feet. Remain springy in your step. This will greatly increase the positive effect and it will prevent injuries. Here's what to do, step by step:

* Perform four 5-minute intervals.

* Start by raising ramp all the way up to 15.

* Keep your speed anywhere from 3.0 to 4.0, depending on your athletic ability and height. If you haven't worked out much, start at 3.0. Taller women (over five foot seven), who tend to have a longer stride, can begin in the upper range of 4.0. Walk at your speed for 2 minutes.

* Then lower the ramp to 1.0 and jog for 2 minutes at a speed of 4.5 to 6.5, depending on your height and ability.

* Lower your speed and your ramp to 3.5 or to comfortable walking speed for 1 minute.

* Repeat this interval 3 more times to equal a total of 20 minutes.

* Every other day of the cardio routine, try to increase your speed on both the uphill portion and the flat run. I started walking at 3.8 and running at 6.0, for example. I now walk at 4.5 and run at 8.0. As your body adapts, your goal should be speed, not time.

The Elliptical Program

Elliptical trainers are a cross between stair-steppers and treadmills. The smooth motion of an elliptical means less impact on the lower body (which is important for people with joint problems) because your foot never leaves the pedal. If used correctly, elliptical trainers are super calorie burners. Make sure not to relax your joints or muscles while pedaling. As with any machine, don't lean on it. Keep your body upright with your hands lightly touching the machine. Leaning heavily on the handlebars only decreases how hard your legs must work, and you won't get a good calorie burn. Here's what to do, step by step:

* Perform four 5-minute intervals.

* Lower the cross ramp between 1 and 5. Keep your resistance at a pace that allows you to pedal fast and hard. Try to keep it above 170 strides per minute. Do this for 2 minutes.

* For the next 2 minutes, raise the cross ramp as high as it will go, increasing your resistance so that you are struggling to move your legs against it.

* For 1 minute, lower the ramp to between 1 and 5 and decrease your resistance so you can pedal at a comfortable pace.

* Repeat this interval 3 more times to equal a total of 20 minutes.

Each day that you do the cardio program, try to up your intensity, increasing the resistance on the flat ramp and pedaling faster.

The Stair-Climber Program

A stair-climber is one of the best forms of cardio. I never sweat so much as I do on the stair-climber. I especially love how it targets my butt and lifts it, as well as shapes my calves, so if your gym has one of these, use it. The way to get intensity with this machine is by increasing speed, skipping steps, or walking sideways. Here's what to do:

* Perform two 10-minute segments.

* Start off at a reasonable speed, such as 70 steps per minute. For the first 4 minutes, take each step, one by one. Try not to hold on to the side rail.

* For the next 4 minutes, skip a step. Really focus on your butt and the backs of your legs. Try to push off with your heel, not your toes. Keep your back straight, chest out, and shoulders back. You can lightly touch handrails for balance.

* Step for 1 minute at a slower speed, such as 60 steps per minute.

* Repeat this interval 1 more time.

In week 2 of your stair-stepping program, increase your speed. For example:

* Perform two 10-minute intervals.

* Start off at a reasonable speed, such as 90 steps per minute. For the first 4 minutes, take each step one by one. Try not to hold on to the side rail.

* For the next 4 minutes at 90 steps a minute, skip a step.

* Step for 1 minute at 70 steps per minute.

* Repeat this interval 1 more time.

The Walking/Hiking Program

If you don't have access to any gym equipment, I suggest you start an outdoor walk/run program. Find a neighborhood that has some hills and wear a watch to time yourself. Invest in a pedometer to track your progress and increase each day. As with the treadmill, keep your body tight and do not slap down your feet. Run with a spring in your step, look forward, and keep your chest out and shoulders back. Walking and running outdoors is not only a beautiful experience, but also challenges your leg muscles and your cardiovascular system, making it a significant calorie burner and leg toner. Going up and down inclines is hard work, and unpaved trails and steep grades also engage your core muscles as you negotiate uneven ground. Here's what to do:

* Perform four 5-minute intervals.

* For 2 minutes, walk/lunge at a fast pace, bringing each knee close to the ground and taking deep, wide steps.

* For the next 2 minutes, jog as fast as you can without stopping.

* For 1 minute, walk casually.

* Repeat this interval 3 more times to equal 20 minutes.

* In week 2, try to increase your walking and jogging pace. Another way to increase your intensity is to vary your location by finding a hilly trail to run on.

The Indoor Biking Program

Stationary bikes are very popular, but are rarely used intensely. Riding a stationary bike works your lower body and core. As with the elliptical trainer, you can increase resistance, thereby increasing muscle tone. Here's what to do:

* Perform four 5-minute intervals.

* For 2 minutes, pedal at a resistance that feels challenging (usually about 30 percent of maximum) but still lets you go at a very fast pace. Keep your muscles tight and engage your core.

* For the next 2 minutes, increase your resistance to about 70 percent of maximum and stand up on your bike. Pedal hard on this interval. By "hard," I mean you should feel like you're pedaling through mud. This action will really work your core, too.

* For 1 minute, pedal at a comfortable pace at a resistance that is about 50 percent of maximum.

* Repeat this interval 3 more times for a total of 20 minutes. Keep your shoulders down and back, and don't hunch over the handlebars.

In week 2, increase your resistance. For example:

* Perform four 5-minute intervals.

* For 2 minutes, pedal fast at a 40 percent resistance.

* For the next 2 minutes, increase your resistance to about 80 percent of maximum and stand up on your bike. Pedal hard on this interval, like you're pedaling through mud.

* For 1 minute, pedal at a comfortable pace and a resistance that's about 50 percent of maximum.

* Repeat these intervals 3 more times for a total of 20 minutes, using good form.

In time, you can change the program up by switching the order. On some days, stand out of your seat and pedal fast for 2 minutes, then sit in the seat and increase resistance for 2 minutes.

The Swimming Program

Swimming is often considered the best all-around exercise. The rhythmic movements involved in pounding through the water work all your major muscle groups, as well as the heart and lungs. Swimming is excellent for building muscle strength and endurance and is easy on the joints, which is why it's often recommended for those suffering from back or mobility problems. Also, swimming is especially good for conditioning the muscles of the upper body because of the effort needed to propel the body through the water. Therefore, it's a great choice if you want to develop your chest and abdominal muscles while improving your aerobic capacity.

An intense twenty-minute cardio swim is easy to organize. Here's how:

* Perform four 5-minute intervals.

* For the first 4 minutes, swim at a brisk, consistent pace.

* For 1 minute, swim at a slower pace.

* Repeat the interval 3 more times for a total of 20 minutes.

* To fight possible boredom, change your stroke every 4-minute interval.

Prepping Your Body

Do my two-week twenty-minute cardio routine during the same two weeks you're adding food in. Both programs prep your body for the workout to come. You'll start losing weight and toning your body with both two-week programs. Plus, you'll feel so much stronger and ready to take it to the next level after these two weeks.

That's when you'll add resistance training to the mix, but not your ordinary weight-lifting moves. I've created and tested countless moves, with one objective in mind: to help you get your fittest, sexiest body ever. Most of these moves use nothing but your own body weight or a set of dumbbells—which means you can do them anywhere, anytime. They're mostly exercises you've never done before, and I know you'll actually enjoy them once you get started. But best of all, they'll shape and tighten your body, develop body-slimming muscle tissue, and give you a firmer, more defined look. Let's get started.

8 Building the Perfect Machine

I'm going to say it again and again—muscle is the quickest way to a hot, healthy body. If you just go on a diet, or if you just diet and do aerobics, you may end up a little thinner, but unfortunately, you'd have to work so much harder to keep your weight down. Muscle is the only thing that speeds up your metabolism so that you can consistently burn calories for hours and while resting. So for any noticeable body change, you need to develop muscle, and you do that through resistance training. This means using weights, your own body weight, or sculpting tools like exercise bands in your workout.

I hear time and again from women who are afraid to lift weights. Instead, they gravitate to aerobic-type exercise because they're afraid they'll look "thick." Relax. Women have less muscle mass than men because they have less testosterone and fewer of the cells that make up muscle fiber. My program is designed to help you get the best out of your genetic body type by decreasing your fat and increasing your tone. When this happens, you lose inches, too, because muscle is dense and compact, while fat is loose and makes your figure look like jelly. So throw away all your old conceptions about resistance training, and let me re-inspire you. Start looking to the Nike models, not the supermodels, for inspiration. Skinny fat is out and sexy tone is the hot new look of today. Resistance training is the quickest way to your sexiest body.

Muscle Matters

If you push yourself with a good, intense resistance-training program, your muscles will respond. Not only will the pounds start dropping, but you'll completely change your body shape for the better. You'll lose fat thighs, flabby arms, and soft bellies. Your skin will appear firmer, too, and your bones and ligaments will become stronger.

The more lean muscle you have on your body, the more your metabolism rises. It is estimated that one pound of muscle requires fifty to a hundred calories per day to function. Increasing your lean muscle by as little as three to five pounds can have a profound effect on your daily caloric burn by raising your basal metabolic rate (BMR), which is the number of calories you expend while sitting or sleeping. So if you add three to five pounds of muscle to your body, your BMR will increase by 250 to 500 calories per day. If you maintain or

FAT-BURNING FACT: FEEL THE AFTERBURN WITH RESISTANCE TRAINING

AFTER YOUR RESISTANCE-TRAINING workout, your body benefits from the afterburn—the calories your body continues to burn long after you leave the gym. A study conducted at Ohio University found that the afterburn can last up to thirty-eight hours. That's like getting the calorie-burning benefit of extra workouts! The exercisers in the study, incidentally, worked out using a thirty-minute circuit routine, which is the type of training I advocate. When you finish exercising, areas of the body that are oxygen-deficient work to recover what they loaned to the muscles. Your body also works to restore hormone balance and to cool down. All of that requires oxygen, and the afterburn occurs until your body restores itself. To maximize your afterburn, step out of your comfort zone. The more intense your effort, the better and faster your results.

Source: European Journal of Applied Physiology

decrease your calorie intake, that's equivalent to one to three pounds of fat loss per week.

Great trainers know the importance of muscle. Many of us are able to eat whatever we want—not because of exceptional genetics, but because of muscle. So the more muscle, the more allowances in food you can eventually give yourself, or at least your battle to get thin will be so much easier.

I'd like to emphasize that starting this workout program is not an excuse to pig out. Why would you spend hours burning off calories just to pile them back on? The goal is to be calorie-deficient each week, and exercising makes that happen. If you're eating like a pig on workout days or rewarding yourself with too much food after every workout, you'll be breaking even and not seeing strong results. If you burned five hundred calories during your workout, for example, then allow yourself a splurge or help yourself to second helpings at dinner every time, you're wasting time and effort. When I feel tempted to overeat, I think to myself: *Eating this cake means I have to triple my cardio tomorrow.* That usually does the trick, because I hate cardio! Don't blow your workouts with bad snacks.

Resistance training also changes the hormonal environment in your body—for the better. Two of the major fat-burning hormones, testosterone and growth hormone—which assist in building muscle and eliminating fat—skyrocket during your exercise sessions. Afterward, DHEA kicks in. DHEA is an amazing hormone, responsible for fat burning, muscle building, mood, sex drive, and immunity. Supplies dwindle with age, so do everything you can to keep levels high, including exercise.

> ## FAT-BURNING FACT: RESISTANCE TRAINING BURNS FAT
>
> **MOST PEOPLE BELIEVE** that if you want to burn the most fat, you should do lots of cardio. Well, it's time to throw this dated assumption out. Resistance training is the best way to get rid of fat—better than dieting alone or even dieting and doing aerobic exercise. Research shows that people who diet but don't exercise lose 69 percent of their fat; people who diet and do aerobic exercise lose 78 percent of their fat; and *those who diet, do aerobics, and lift weights burn 97 percent of their fat.*
>
> *Source: Ball State University*

Home or Gym?

Maybe you're wondering: *Do I have to join a gym to do this workout program, or can I do it at home?*

You can absolutely do this workout at home, and not a lot of equipment is needed. You'll want to invest in an exercise mat and two sets of dumbbells. One set should be lighter in weight (between three and eight pounds) and the other should be heavier (between twelve and fifteen pounds). Most of my exercises use the resistance of your own body weight, which is why you don't need to buy much equipment.

There are advantages to being able to work out at home. You save a lot of excess time if you don't have to drive. You can just walk into any room of your house you've designated as your workout area, and do your exercises. And you have complete privacy. My exercises can also be done in a hotel room, so you never have to miss a workout while on the road.

Of course, if you're someone who likes the gym atmosphere, you can definitely do my program at a gym. There are lots of pluses to joining a gym. The people you meet there can be a very positive force in your life. They're great role models who can provide an excellent support system. So if you join a gym, make friends with other members. It's inspiring to be around people who are trying to accomplish the same goals you are.

> ### HEALTHY PEOPLE HAVE HOTTER SEX!
>
> **SOMETIMES IN LIFE** you have to face some ugly truths. One truth is that being fat isn't good for your love life. If you're looking to attract men, then you should know they just aren't crazy about an overweight mate, according to a survey of twenty-seven thousand men and women conducted by *Elle* magazine and MSNBC in 2006. More than 31 percent of men said they had dumped a partner who was overweight, compared with 12 percent of women. If you want to get dates, get thin!

Gym Etiquette

If anybody knows about proper gym etiquette, it's me. I own a gym and have to constantly stay on top of my staff to follow the rules. A lot of clients tell me that they're intimidated by gyms because they feel they don't know how to use the equipment or feel they are out of place, in the way. Part of feeling comfortable in the gym is knowing the rules of a gym. I'll clear up a few of these for you, so you can go into any gym with confidence.

* Learn the proper operation of equipment. If you're unsure of how something works, ask for assistance.

* Pick up after yourself. Put your weights away. The next people in line don't want to hunt around for the weights they need or, worse yet, try to remove the weights you left out.

* Allow people to "work in." Many people do multiple sets on the weight machines, then sit on the equipment during their recovery time. If someone is waiting to use the same machine, the proper etiquette is to allow her to work in or do her set while you recover. So do your set, get off, and let the other person work in. Don't be shy about asking someone if you can work in, either. However, don't work in if there are already two people waiting to use the same equipment.

* Don't drop weights. Not only is dropping weights dangerous for your toes, but it damages the equipment and the floor. The rule of thumb is: If you can lift it, you can put it down gently.

* Observe time limits on cardio equipment. Some gyms have time limits (usually thirty minutes) on the cardio equipment (treadmills, elliptical trainers, stationary bikes, and so on), especially during peak hours. If you see people waiting around to use your type of machine, be especially conscious of the time limit.

* Wipe your sweat off the equipment. Gyms are notorious places for spreading nasty germs like staph infections, so practice good hygiene. And always lay a towel on the equipment to protect yourself.

* Don't disturb other gymgoers. The gym can be a great place to meet other healthy people. But don't be too chatty. You are there to work to intensity. Stay focused on your goals.

Workout Lingo

If you're going to do my program, you've got to be familiar with the workout language spoken. A quick read-through of the following terms, and you'll be fluent.

* *Rep.* One complete motion of an exercise from starting position back to starting position.

* *Sets.* The specific number of reps you perform on one exercise.

* *Form.* The correct technique involved in performing an exercise. This typically involves proper posture and control of reps. A common mistake among exercisers is to do reps with rapid, jerky movements. This adds no real resistance and can actually damage your joints. Without resistance, muscles aren't properly challenged and won't respond as well.

* *Routine.* The complete series of exercises that you perform during your workout. A whole-body routine can be done in one session and repeated several times per week. Other routines are "split routines," in which you work certain body parts like chest and triceps in one workout; legs and abs in another; and back, biceps, and shoulders in a third, with each body-part workout done on a different day.

* *Circuit routine.* This is a routine in which you perform numerous exercises back-to-back with little rest in between. An example is my Power Circuit training routine, which I'll cover in chapter 10. One reason circuit training is so effective is that it targets more of your muscle fibers. This will help you burn more fat and get more definition.

* *Contraction.* Squeezing or tightening the muscle you are working.

*   *Resistance.* The challenge (in the form of weights, resistance bands, or your own body weight) applied to muscular contraction.

*   *Failure.* When you can no longer do another rep in good form. Your muscles have been exhausted.

*   *Rest.* The time taken either between exercise sets or between workouts. Rest is necessary for muscle to repair and rebuild. During a workout, it takes one minute for your body to replenish muscle energy (technically known as ATP). In my routines, you rest your upper body while working your lower. That way, muscle energy is still being replaced, so you don't have to slow down the pace of your workout. After a workout, allow the muscles you worked to rest for forty-eight hours. Don't rest longer than two days, however. After two days of inactivity, less glucose is taken into your muscles as energy and is instead packed away as fat.

*   *Breathing.* In resistance training, breathing means inhaling during the lifting phase and exhaling with the return movement. Make sure not to hold your breath during an exercise or you may become dizzy. When you hold your breath too long, blood flow to the head slows down, reducing the supply of oxygen to the brain.

*   *Frequency.* How often you work out during the week. On my program, you'll do Power Circuits three times a week, and cardio five times a week.

*   *Duration.* How long your particular workout lasts. I believe in thirty-minute resistance routines that are very intense and twenty-minute cardio routines performed prior to resistance training.

Do You Need a Personal Trainer?

You can do my program with or without a personal trainer. The advantage of working with a trainer is that he or she can keep you from plateauing, make you accountable, and push you harder than you can push yourself. When thinking about hiring a personal trainer, watch for these things:

* *Certifications.* Look for certification from one of the major health and fitness organizations. These include National Academy of Sports Medicine (NASM), the National Council on Strength and Fitness (NCSF), the American Council on Exercise (ACE), the Aerobics and Fitness Association of America (AFAA), the International Sports Sciences Association (ISSA), the National Federation of Professional Trainers (NFPT), the American Fitness Training of Athletics (AFTA), the National Exercise & Sports Trainers Association (NESTA), the International Fitness Professionals Association (IFPA), and the American Fitness Institute (AFI). Also, ask about their background and length of experience, and whether they're certified in cardiopulmonary resuscitation and first aid. (Most certifications require CPR training, but it's good to check anyway.)

* *Experience.* Ask how many years of experience a personal trainer has working with clients. Does he or she have expertise in a certain area of fitness that you enjoy or would like to learn? If you've always wanted to learn how to box, for example, make sure your trainer has the expertise to incorporate some boxing moves into your routine. A trainer should know your exercise history, injuries, training goals, and any pain you might have—and design sessions that account for this. If you are under the care of a medical or orthopedic physician, your personal trainer should also ask the doctor for medical clearance.

* *Gender.* I'm a strong believer that women should train women and men should train men. Women know another woman's pain threshold and will not listen to whining and excuses. In my experience, men let a female client off the hook too easily the moment she complains. Of course, there are exceptions to this rule. The

most important thing is that you get a knowledgeable and experienced personal trainer who fits your style—because that is the professional who will help you achieve the best results.

* *Cost.* Decide how much you're willing to spend and allow for that budget for at least three months. This will give you motivation and time to achieve your goals. Trainers can cost anywhere from twenty-five to two hundred dollars an hour or more, depending on their professional background, clientele, and services.

* *Personality.* Developing a personal yet professional relationship with your trainer is very important. Trust your instincts. Ask yourself if you think your trainer is willing to work hard with you. A personal trainer should be passionate and be willing to teach you how to empower yourself. Remember, your trainer is your life coach, not your friend. It never ends well when trainers and clients socialize too much together, because your workouts become chatty and less effective. Remember, it should be all about you! Many times, a personal trainer takes on the role of a therapist and should maintain that professional relationship.

* *References.* When possible, always talk to gym owners or managers about whom they would recommend for you, based on your goals and interests.

Now you're ready to learn my exercises. I'm not going to give you the same old, boring exercises you've read about in every other fitness book. Take it from someone who has trained for more than twenty years: Variety is the key to success, especially with exercise. You can't get consistent results if you're bored. I don't want you to be bored, so I've come up with a challenging program to which your body will quickly respond.

9 My Fat-Burning Exercises

Over the next several pages, you'll find step-by-step instructions on how to perform all my exercises. Every movement is carefully illustrated with photographs to show you what proper form and technique look like and text that explains how to achieve it. Read through each exercise; then practice it. Go slowly in order to master it.

Very important: Use proper form. Learn to feel every exercise you're doing. The more you're in touch with your working muscles while exercising, the more profound your results will be. This is called the mind-muscle connection. It involves visualizing and focusing on the muscle as it contracts during an exercise. For example, as you work your abs, you visualize and feel the muscles working while you move through the exercise. The improved focus actually leads to better growth.

Researchers from Hull University in the United Kingdom put this to the test. They asked exercisers to perform biceps curls under two different conditions while the muscle activity of the biceps was measured. In one trial, subjects did biceps curls while focusing on the biceps and the act of performing the curls. In another trial, the subjects did curls while focusing just on lifting the weight, not on the muscle. The scientists found that when the exercisers focused on the actual muscle, more muscle fibers were activated compared with when they focused on just the weight. These findings mean the mind-muscle connection is the real deal. It can help you increase the number of muscle fibers you utilize, which in turn will enhance muscle tone and development. You know what that leads to—a fat-burning body!

My Warm-Up Exercises

Most people know they should warm up before starting their workouts, yet they want to skip it. A good warm-up:

* Generates more muscle force so you can work out harder and burn more fat.

* Helps you focus and prepare for the workout ahead.

* Increases blood flow to the working muscles. More blood means more oxygen and nutrients to fuel exercise, and efficient removal of metabolic by-products such as lactic acid. Increased blood flow also protects you against injuries.

* Lubricates your joints for easier movement and adjusts the levels of hormones responsible for energy production. In other words, you "get your juices flowing."

Here are my favorite warm-up exercises. Do them each for thirty seconds prior to your Power Circuit, and you'll be ready to go. (Remember that before beginning this or any workout program, you should consult your physician or health-care professional.)

CHAIN BREAKERS

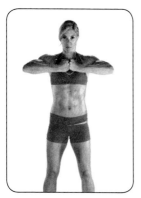

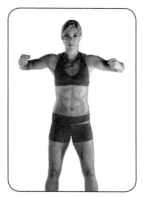

Stand with your feet about 6 inches apart. Bring your arms up with clenched fists at chest level.

With elbows locked in a bent position, open and shut your arms quickly while keeping your elbows at chest level.

KNEE-UPS

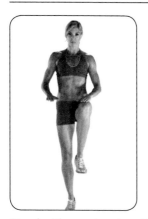

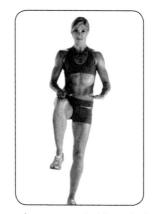

Stand with your legs together and your arms held out in front of you. Lift your left knee up so that it is parallel to the floor. Lower your left leg back to the floor. Repeat the move with your right knee. Alternate the knee-ups for 30 seconds.

Jumping Jacks

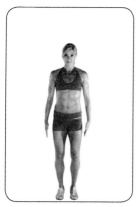 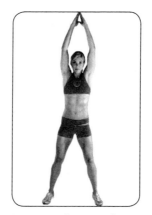

Start with your feet about a foot apart and hands at your sides. Keep your back straight. Bend your knees slightly.

Jump, moving your feet apart until they are wider than your shoulders. At the same time, raise your arms over your head. You should be on the balls of your feet.

Jump again, bringing your feet together and your arms back to your sides. At the end of the movement, your weight should be on your heels.

Shoulder Crossovers

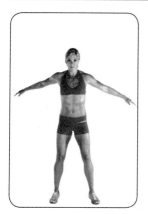 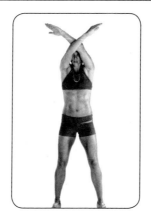

Straighten your arms and cross them in front of and above your head, then open wide.

HEAD ROLLS

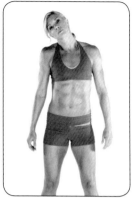

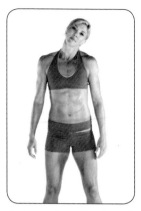

Stand straight, with your feet about 6 inches apart. Roll your right ear to your right shoulder.

Roll your head back. Roll your left ear to your left shoulder. Roll your chin back to your chest.

My Exercises

Hamstring Exercises

DUMBBELL DEAD LIFTS

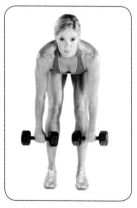

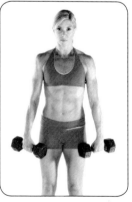

Holding two dumbbells in front of you, slowly bend down from your back to the point of reaching just below your knees. Keep your back slightly arched.

Come back up to the starting position, squeezing your butt.

Keep your abs tight and your knees slightly bent but locked.

Perform 15 repetitions for 3 sets.

CROSS-KNEE BRIDGES

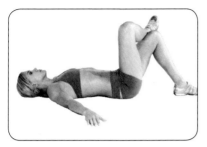
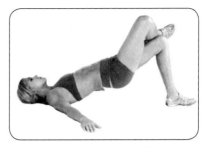

Lie on your back on an exercise mat, with your arms at your sides. Rest your right foot on your left knee.

Slowly lift your pelvis up off the mat until your back is flat. Hold and return to the starting position.

Perform 15 repetitions each leg for 3 sets.

ALTERNATE SPLIT JUMPS

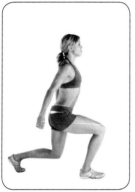
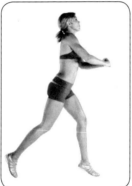

Begin in a lunge position with your legs straddled about a stride's length apart, left foot forward, with both knees bent so that your left thigh is parallel to the ground and your right knee is nearly touching it, heel lifted.

Jump up and scissor your legs quickly so your legs (as well as your arms) switch places. Control your movements and keep your head and torso movement to a minimum. Land springy. Continue to alternate right and left scissor jumps.

Perform 20 total repetitions for 3 sets.

REVERSE PLANKS

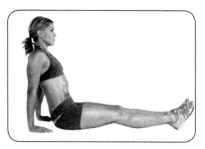 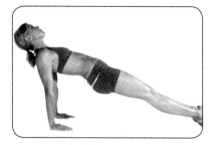

Sit down on an exercise mat with your legs stretched out in front of you. Place your arms behind you with your hands palms down on the mat and your fingers pointing forward. Keep your hands flat.

Press your body up using your arms. Lift your hips up toward the ceiling. Don't let your torso sag, but instead maintain a straight line from your shoulders to the heels of your feet. Then drop your butt down toward the floor but not touching. Repeat the lift.

Perform 15 repetitions for 3 sets.

Quadriceps Exercises

UFCs

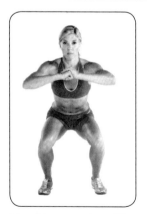 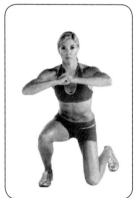 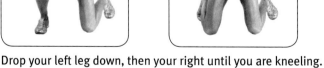

Stand in a squat position. Keep your back straight and your abs engaged.

Drop your left leg down, then your right until you are kneeling.

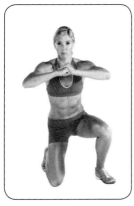

Return your left leg to its starting position and repeat the action on your right leg, always returning to the squat position.

Perform 30 total repetitions for 3 sets.

FRONT KICKS

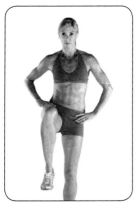
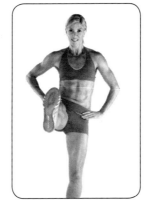

Stand with your feet flat on the floor. Raise one leg toward your stomach as high as you can.

Then kick out from your knee—but don't drop your leg down.

Bring your leg back in toward your stomach and return to the starting position. Repeat with the other leg.

Perform 15 repetitions on each leg for 3 sets.

SISSY SQUATS

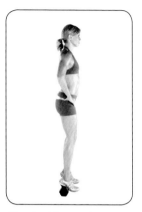 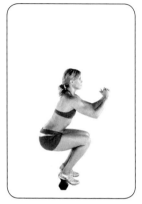

Stand with your legs shoulder-width apart and your heels on your dumbbells.

Squat down until your knees are parallel to the floor. Pause at the bottom for a second or two. Return to the starting position and repeat the movement until you have completed a full set.

Perform 15 repetitions for 3 sets.

FRONT DUMBBELL LUNGES

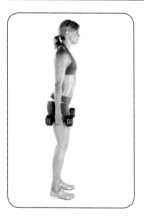 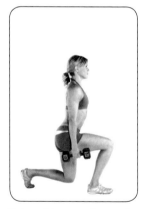

Begin with your feet together, your chest out, and your shoulders back. Hold a dumbbell in each hand at your sides.

Take a big step forward on your right foot and lower the opposite knee to the ground. Then push back to the starting position without bouncing. Make sure you put your weight on the lunging heel, not on your toe.

Repeat the movement until you have completed a full set on each leg.

Perform 15 repetitions on each leg for 3 sets.

JUMP SQUATS

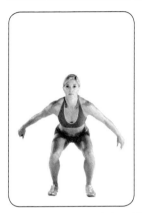

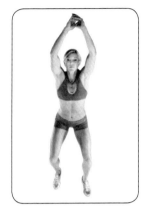

With your feet slightly wider than shoulder-width apart, squat as if you were about to sit on a chair. Your toes should be pointed straight ahead.

Push off your feet to explode upward into a jump. Repeat the movement until you have completed a full set.

Perform 20 repetitions for 3 sets.

Glute (Buttocks) Exercises

DUMBBELL FRONT SQUATS

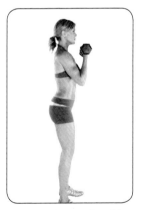

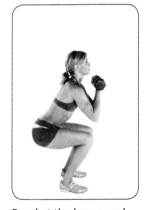

Stand with your feet hip-width apart, your knees slightly bent, and your toes pointing forward. Hold dumbbells in front of your chest.

Bend at the knees and lower your body as if you were going to sit in a chair. Your thighs should be about parallel to the floor.

Straighten your legs to return to the starting position, pressing back up from your heels.

Perform 15 repetitions for 3 sets.

BACK BRIDGES

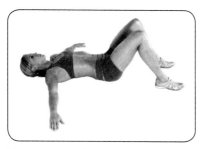 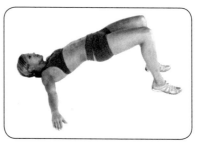

Lie on an exercise mat with your knees bent and your arms out to your sides.

Press into the floor with your feet, contract your buttocks and abdominals, and raise your hips off the floor until your body forms a diagonal line. Lower 1 inch from the floor, never relaxing. Concentrate on squeezing your glutes throughout the move.

Perform 15 repetitions for 3 sets.

HEISMANS

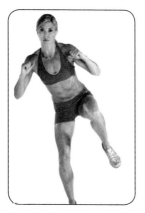 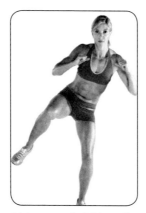

Stand with your feet shoulder-width apart. Quickly pull one knee up and across the front of your body toward your opposing hand. Keep your torso pointed straight forward.

Jump from side to side, always tucking your knee up toward your torso.

Alternate sides for a total of 30 repetitions for 3 sets.

SUMO SQUATS

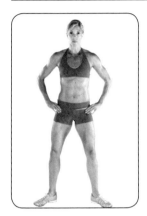
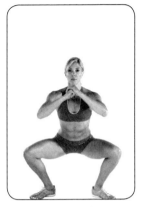

Stand with your feet wider apart than shoulder-width, as shown. Turn your toes out about 45 degrees. Keep your shoulders back and your hips tucked.

Slowly bend at the knees and lower your body until your hamstrings are parallel to the floor.

Pause for a second in the bottom position; then push up through your heels to drive back up to the starting position.

Perform 15 repetitions for 3 sets.

DONKEY-KICK CROSSOVERS

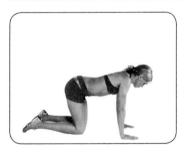
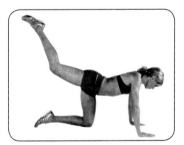

Begin on all fours (hands under your shoulders, knees under your hips).

Lift your right leg up above hip level and flex your right knee. Extend your leg upward as high as you can go.

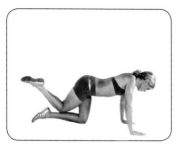

Lower your right knee and cross it over the back of your left knee.

Return your right leg to the starting position. Complete a full set with the right leg. Switch legs and repeat the exercise with the left leg.

Perform a total of 30 repetitions for 3 sets.

Chest Exercises

DUMBBELL PRESSES WITH TWIST

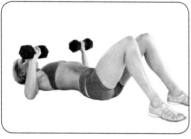 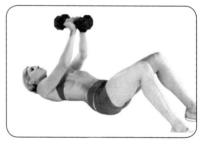

Lie on your back on the floor or exercise mat, knees bent and feet flat on the floor or mat. Hold a dumbbell in each hand just above your chest, palms facing forward.

Then slowly bend your elbows, lowering the weights down and to your sides until your arms form a 90-degree angle, elbows in line with your shoulders.

Raise the dumbbells toward the ceiling, simultaneously turning your forearms so that your palms now face you.

Perform 15 repetitions for 3 sets.

DUMBBELL FLYES

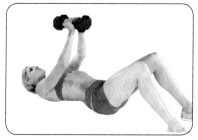

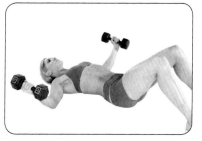

Hold a dumbbell in each hand and lie back on the floor or an exercise mat.

With your palms facing each other, extend your arms straight up so that the dumbbells are directly over your chest.

Slightly bend your elbows and extend them downward in an arc until you feel a complete stretch in your upper chest. Hold the open position for a pause.

Now squeeze your chest muscles and draw your arms back to the starting position.

Perform 15 repetitions for 3 sets.

DUMBBELL HAMMER PRESSES

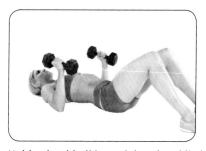

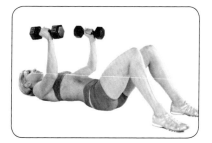

Hold a dumbbell in each hand and lie back on the floor or an exercise mat. Hold the dumbbells at chest level so that the end of the weights are pointed vertically toward your head, as shown. The palms of your hands should be facing each other.

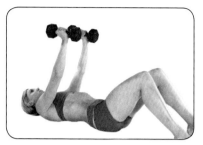

Extend your arms overhead. Slowly lower the weights back to the starting position.

Perform 15 repetitions for 3 sets.

REVERSE DUMBBELL PRESSES

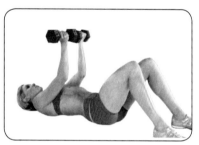

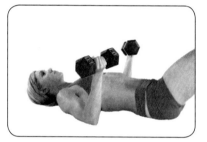

Hold a dumbbell in each hand with a reverse grip so that your palms are facing your face. Hold the weights just above your chest, arms straight but not locked.

Then slowly bend your elbows, lowering the weights down and to your sides until your arms form a 90-degree angle, your elbows in line with your shoulders.

Raise the weights to the starting position.

Perform 15 repetitions for 3 sets.

RENEGADE PUSH-UPS

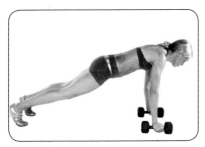

Place two dumbbells on the floor about shoulder-width apart. Grip the dumbbells firmly with your body in a push-up position.

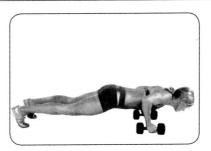

Lower down to floor and push up.

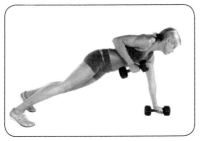

Place all your body weight on your left arm as you pick the right dumbbell off the floor and lift in a rowing motion.

Lower the dumbbell to the floor as you dip into a push-up position. Use your feet to help you balance. Return to the position in which you are gripping both dumbbells.

Put all your weight on your right side as you lift the left dumbbell with your left hand. Drop to your knees if you need to modify. Continue to alternate from side to side for a total of 30 repetitions.

Back Exercises

WIDE DUMBBELL PULLS

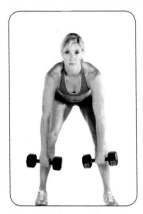

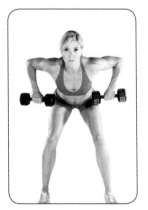

Stand with your feet about shoulder-width apart. Grasp a dumbbell in each hand. Bend forward at the waist until your back is almost parallel to the floor. Keep a slight arch in your back.

Keep your arms fully extended, several inches out from your sides, and palms facing inward. Lift the weights up to your sides until you can lift no higher.

Lower the weights slowly to the starting position.

Perform 15 repetitions for 3 sets.

WINGMANS

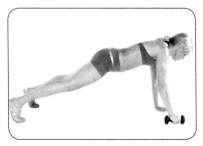

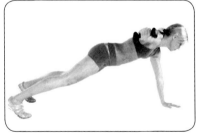

Put your body in the plank position, as shown. Grip a dumbbell in your right hand, as shown. Keep your back straight.

Lift the right dumbbell straight out to your side in a controlled fashion.

Lower it slowly to the starting position.

Repeat the exercise on the left side.

Alternate for 30 total repetitions for 3 sets.

ALTERNATING DUMBBELL ROWS

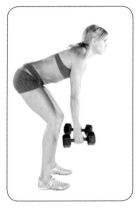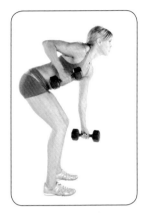

Lean forward so that your torso is at about a 45-degree angle to the floor.

Hold a dumbbell in each hand, palms toward your body, arms straight. Raise the right dumbbell by pulling your arm up and toward your spine, bringing your elbow as high as you can. Squeeze your back muscles briefly at the top and lower the weight along the same path.

Repeat with your left arm. Alternate right and left arms for a total of 30 repetitions.

SWIMMERS

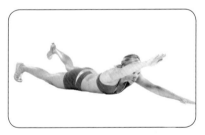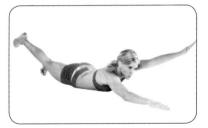

Lie facedown on the floor or an exercise mat with your hands outstretched, as shown. Bring your right arm and your left leg up simultaneously. Hold them there as you lift your head and chest off the mat.

Switch your arms and legs by lifting your left arm and right leg above the floor. Squeeze your butt as you do this exercise.

Continue switching pairs in this manner as though you are performing a swimming motion.

Perform 30 repetitions for 3 sets.

DUMBBELL PULLOVERS

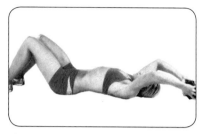 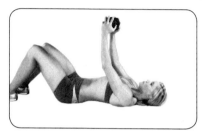

Lie on your back on the floor or an exercise mat. Hold the ends of one dumbbell in both hands, your arms extended behind you, elbows slightly bent.

Squeeze your shoulder blades together and bring the dumbbell up and over your chest. Contract your back muscles to lift the weight back up.

Repeat the movement until you have completed a full set.

Perform 15 repetitions for 3 sets.

Biceps Exercises

CONCENTRATION CURLS

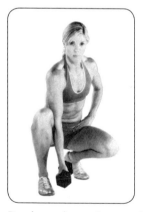 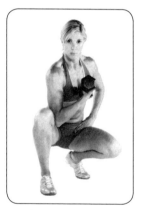

Bend your knees to a semi-squat position, as shown. Hold a dumbbell in your right hand. Let your arm hang down in line with your shoulder, palm facing outward. Place your left hand on your left thigh for support.

Bend your right elbow to curl the dumbbell toward your left shoulder. Slowly lower and repeat the movement until you have completed a full set, then switch arms.

Perform 15 repetitions on each arm for 3 sets.

ALTERNATING DUMBBELL CURLS WITH ROTATION

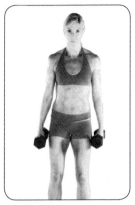
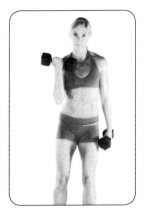
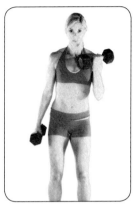

From a standing position, hold a dumbbell in each hand with your arms at your sides. Your palms should be facing your body.

Curl one dumbbell up to shoulder height, rotating your arm so that your palm faces upward.

Lower slowly and repeat with the other arm.

Repeat the movement until you have completed a full set.

Perform 30 total repetitions for 3 sets.

OUTER CURLS

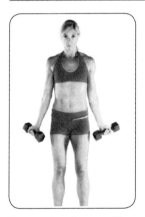
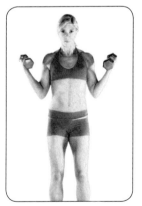

From a standing position, grasp a dumbbell in each hand. Hold your lower arms out at your sides, making sure your palms are facing upward and pointed slightly away from your thighs.

Keeping your upper arms close to your sides, curl the weights upward until you can't bend farther and squeeze the muscles at the top of the contraction. Lower slowly and repeat the movement.

Perform 15 repetitions for 3 sets.

HAMMER CURLS

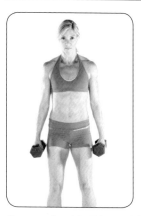 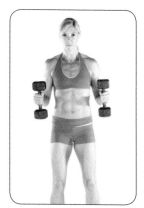

Grasp a dumbbell in each hand and stand with your arms hanging at your sides, palms facing inward. Keep your arms close to your sides.

Curl the dumbbells as high as you can go, squeezing your biceps hard at the top of the lift, and then slowly lower. The top of the weights should be pointing toward the ceiling.

Perform 15 repetitions for 3 sets.

REVERSE CURLS

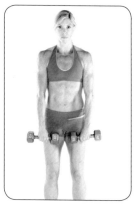 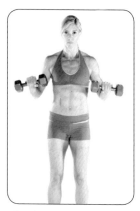

Grasp a dumbbell in each hand and take an overhand grip. Stand with your feet about shoulder-width apart. Let both arms hang down in front of your body, fully extended, with your palms facing in toward your body.

Simultaneously curl the dumbbells upward until you can't bend any farther.

Slowly return to the starting position.

Perform 15 repetitions for 3 sets.

Triceps Exercises

HEADBANGERS

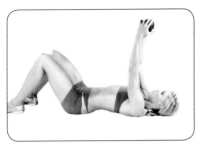 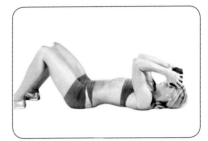

Lie on your back on the floor or an exercise mat. Grasp the ends of one dumbbell with an overhand grip, your palms facing each other.

Hold the dumbbell with straight arms over your forehead, angling your arms back.

Bend your elbows to lower the dumbbell until your forearms are just past parallel with the floor. Let the weights reach just at your forehead.

It is important to not move your upper arms during the lift. The only movement that should occur is the lowering and raising of your forearms.

Perform 15 repetitions for 3 sets.

NARROW PRESSES

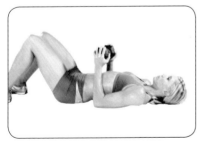

Lie on the floor or an exercise mat and grasp one dumbbell with both hands, with your palms facing each other. Straighten your arms and line them up directly above your chest. This is the starting position.

Keeping elbows close to your sides, push the dumbbell upward to full arm extension.

Without pausing or bouncing at the bottom of the movement, push the dumbbell upward to full arm extension.

Perform 15 repetitions for 3 sets.

KICKBACKS

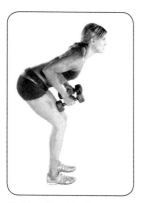 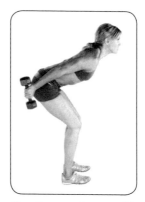

Hold a dumbbell in each hand. Lean over until your torso is at a 45-degree angle to the floor. Bend your elbows and hold your arms against your sides, your palms facing inward.

Simultaneously extend both elbows back so that your arms are in a fully straightened position behind you and in line with your torso.

Reverse the motion to return to the starting position.

Perform 15 repetitions for 3 sets.

NOSE BUSTERS

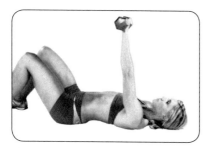 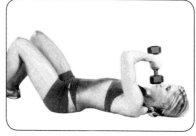

Lie on your back on the floor or an exercise mat. Hold a dumbbell vertically in your left hand at full extension directly over your upper chest.

Without moving your upper arm, bend your elbow to lower the bar to your nose.

Straighten your elbow to drive the weight back to full extension and repeat. Don't let your elbow flare out as you return to the starting position. Perform the exercise with your right arm.

Perform 15 repetitions on each arm for 3 sets.

REVERSE POSTERIOR RAISES

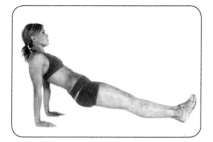

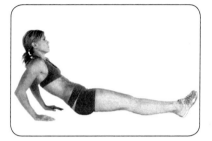

Sit on the floor or exercise mat with your legs fully extended out in front of you. Bring your arms behind you with your palms flat on the mat and your fingers pointing forward. Slowly lift yourself off the ground.

Bend at the elbows until you have lowered your body back to the floor while keeping your arms close to your sides. Straighten your arms to return to the beginning position.

Perform 15 repetitions for 3 sets.

Shoulder Exercises

DUMBBELL LATERAL RAISES

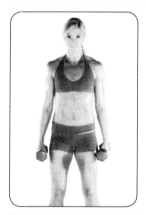

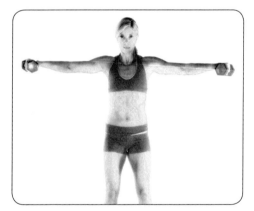

Stand with your feet shoulder-width apart. Grasp a dumbbell in each hand, holding them with your palms facing each other.

Bend your elbows slightly, and raise the dumbbells up and outward until they are slightly higher than shoulder height.

Return to the starting position.

Perform 15 repetitions for 3 sets.

FRONT RAISES

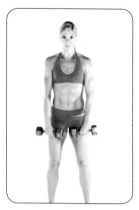

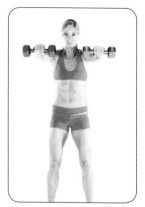

Stand with your feet about shoulder-width apart. Grasp a dumbbell in each hand and hold them across your thighs. Do not lean back as you raise the weights.

Lift the weights upward, your palms facing down and your arms straight out in front, until they are approximately parallel to the floor, then lower them.

Perform 15 repetitions for 3 sets.

BENTOVER REAR FLYES

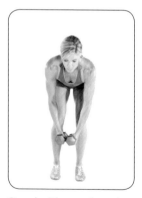

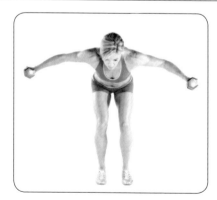

Stand with your feet about shoulder-width apart and your knees slightly bent. Bend forward at your waist. Keep your back straight and your head facing forward. Grasp a dumbbell in each hand with your elbows bent slightly.

Raise your arms outward and upward until the weight reaches shoulder height. Squeeze your shoulder blades together. Return to the starting position.

Perform 15 repetitions for 3 sets.

INS AND OUTS

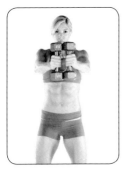

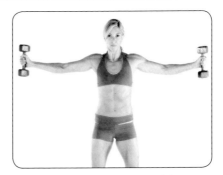

Stand with your feet about shoulder-width apart and your knees slightly bent. Grasp a dumbbell in each hand. Stretch your arms out in front of you, palms facing each other. Your arms should be nearly touching and parallel to the floor.

Open your arms out to your sides.

Return to the starting position.

Perform 15 repetitions for 3 sets.

Ab Exercises

V-TUCKS

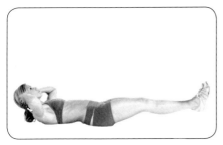

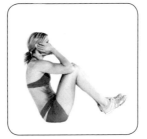

Lie on your back with your hands lightly touching the back of your head. Raise your legs off the floor, as shown.

Bend your knees and tuck them in toward your navel, lifting your torso off the floor. Pause briefly.

Slowly return to the starting position.

Perform 30 repetitions for 3 sets.

BICYCLE

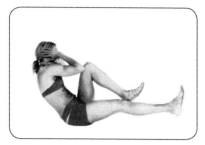

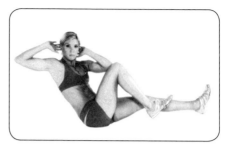

Lie faceup with your fingertips behind your head for light support. Bend your knees, with your feet flat on the floor.

Simultaneously crunch up and cross your right shoulder toward your left knee while pulling that knee in toward your chest. Touch elbow to knee. Alternate from side to side. One touch to each side equals 1 rep.

Perform 30 repetitions for 3 sets.

AB HOLDS

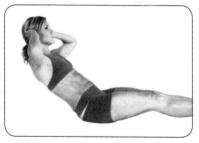

Lie on your back on the floor or an exercise mat with your arms behind your head.

Using the strength of your ab muscles, lift your torso off the floor and hold for 1 minute.

Repeat for 3 total sets.

WINDSHIELD WIPERS

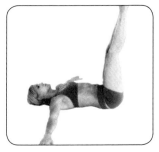 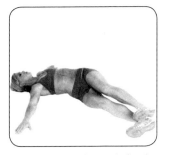 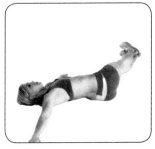

Lie on your back with your feet extended up, so your legs and torso form a 90-degree angle. Your hands should be outstretched to your sides, as shown.

Tighten your abs and slowly drop your legs to the right as far as you can without lifting your shoulder blades from the floor.

Slowly return to the starting position and repeat to the left.

Perform 30 repetitions for 3 sets.

DUMBBELL TRANSVERSES

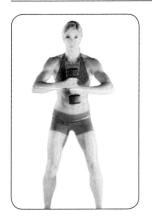 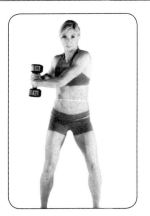

Stand with your feet slightly wider than shoulder-width apart and bend at the knees so that you are in a slight squat position. Grasp one dumbbell with both hands, holding it vertically in front of your torso.

Rotate your torso as far to the right and as far to the left as you can go.

Perform 30 repetitions for 3 sets.

SINGLE-LEG JACKKNIVES

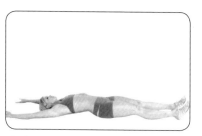

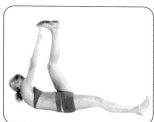

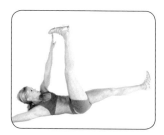

Lie flat on your back with your arms extended straight back behind your head.

Lift your torso, left leg, and right arm simultaneously. Attempt to touch your left toe with your right hand.

Repeat the move with the other arm and leg.

Perform 30 repetitions for 3 total sets.

My Cool-Down Stretches

You'll finish your Power Circuit routine with a series of stretches. This is the cool-down period of your workout. It will help your body recover more quickly and with less muscle soreness. Hold each stretch for thirty seconds without bouncing, and remember to keep breathing.

HURDLER'S STRETCH

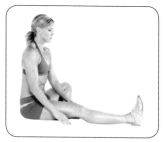

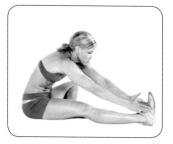

Sit on the floor, with your right leg extended in front of you and your left leg bent and flared out to the side.

Gently bend forward at the hips until you feel a good stretch in your right hamstring. Avoid rounding your back excessively, as this will shift the stretch from your hamstrings to your back. Switch legs.

SUMO STRETCH

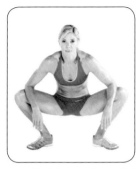

Stand with your feet slightly wider than shoulder-width apart. Point your toes outward. Bend your knees and go into a deep squat. Open your legs by applying pressure with your elbows.

KNEE CROSSOVERS

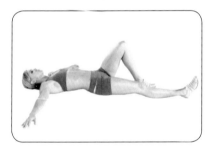 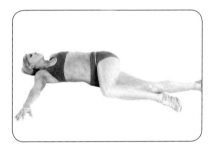

Lie on your back with your arms extended to your sides and your knees bent. Slowly draw your left knee up to your chest, then over your right leg as far as is comfortable. Repeat the move on the other side.

CHEST STRETCH

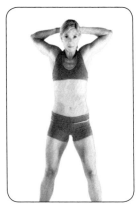

Place your hands behind your head and interlock your fingers. Keep your elbows lifted, as shown. Press your chest forward and your elbows back, getting a good stretch in your chest.

SHOULDER CROSSOVER STRETCH

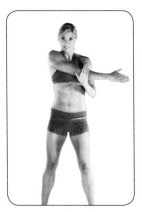

Stand with your feet about shoulder-width apart. Reach your right arm across your chest. Take your other hand and grab the crossed arm's elbow. Press your right arm closer to your body and stretch your shoulder. Repeat the stretch on the other shoulder.

CHILD'S POSE

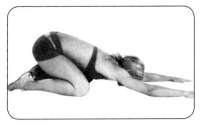

With your toes together, open your knees to at least hip distance apart. Lean forward and drape your body over your thighs so that your forehead rests on the floor. Reach your arms out in front of you. Breathe deeply and relax.

TRICEPS STRETCH

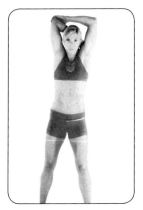 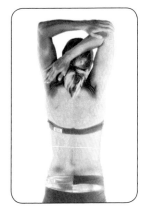

Stand up straight. Keep your knees slightly bent and your abdominal muscles engaged.

Raise your right arm straight overhead. Bend your elbow and place your right palm behind your neck or on the top of your back, wherever you can reach. Maintain a straight spine and neck, and do not push your head forward. With your left hand, tug your right elbow slightly to get a good stretch in your triceps muscle.

Repeat the stretch on the opposite side.

Up Next: Power Circuit Training

In the upcoming chapter, I want to introduce you to a way of working out that I've taught to thousands of clients over the years—Power Circuits. This circuit training format utilizes a group of five resistance-training exercises that are completed one right after the other with very little rest. Along with my diet plan, Power Circuits will help you burn fat faster, develop definition, and give you the body you want.

10 Form, Function, Fatigue

Power Circuits

Everyone is always asking me about the best way to work out to get thin, fit, and toned. They are searching for a magical and easier way to exercise, grasping on to every fad in every magazine. Well, you might be surprised to find out that, yes, there is an ideal, special way to work out that will give you the body you want: Power Circuits. You'll learn how to do them in this chapter.

In This Chapter:

* *The fat-burning benefits of Power Circuit training*
* *Intensity principles for rapid results*
* *Fueling your body before and after exercise*

I'm sure you've heard of "circuit training." Just about everyone has. Circuit training combines the principles of aerobic conditioning and weight lifting to help you burn calories while building strength. It's a popular workout for the time-deprived, and it never gets boring. With circuit training, you work through a series, or circuit, of exercises, completing one right after the other with very little rest between sets. You get the best of both worlds, perfectly combining resistance training (muscle tone/fast metabolism) with cardiovascular activity (calorie loss). The continuous nature of circuit training gives you a major calorie burn. Because there's no rest between sets, you finish your workout in thirty minutes. Further, you can change the exercises in your circuit whenever you want, so there's less chance of falling into an exercise rut.

Some other benefits:

* ***More burn.*** Circuit training simultaneously improves mobility, strength, and stamina and is the best way to burn calories in the fastest time—*period*! This type of exercising has been shown by research to burn more calories in a shorter period of time than conventional exercise routines, thus decreasing body fat. Conventional weight lifting burns 200 to 250 calories an hour, whereas circuit training burns anywhere from 350 to 550. That's a lot more burn for your buck!

* ***More tone.*** Circuit training really tightens and shapes your body. Because many muscles are engaged while circuit training, more toning occurs and more calorie burning occurs.

* ***More smile.*** People who do conventional weight training often miss out on the "runner's high"—that surge of naturally produced endorphins that comes from running, cycling, swimming, and other forms of intense cardio. Endorphins do amazing things: They relieve pain, they reduce stress, they enhance the immune system, and they postpone the aging process. So not only will you look good on the outside, but thanks to circuit training you'll feel good on the inside, too.

Introduction to Power Circuits

All my clients have different goals: Some are getting in shape for the red carpet; others want to make a life change. But one thing they all have in common: They want to lose weight fast—which is why I use my own brand of circuit training called Power Circuits.

Power Circuits are an amped-up version of basic circuit training. You work out harder and faster. It's a constant flow of motion, almost like rowing a boat where you never let the oars stop moving. In addition, Power Circuits alternate between upper- and lower-body exercises, so you don't waste time waiting for all muscle groups to recuperate. With Power Circuits, you're always focusing on large muscle groups like your chest, back, glutes, core, hamstrings, and quadriceps, since they burn the most amount of fat. If you've been working out for a while, but aren't seeing the results you want or have reached a seemingly permanent plateau, Power Circuits will kick-start your body back into results mode.

The 3-F Formula: Form, Function, Fatigue

With my Power Circuits, there's a formula I use to ensure results. I call it my 3-F Formula. This means you combine two *functions* (two exercises) with perfect *form* and do the exercises to complete *fatigue*. And by "fatigue," I mean don't stop till you drop!

I always have my clients work the same muscle group with two different exercises right in a row for more efficient fat burning and a leaner body. An example would be to perform a dumbbell chest press with perfect form until you can barely lift another rep; then you'd quickly do push-ups until you can't press yourself up again. Because you have already fatigued your chest with the dumbbell presses, you'll be able to only do eight to ten push-ups, so it all goes very fast. Muscles respond extremely well to this formula. It's great for reshaping your body fast.

My Intensity Principles

With my Power Circuits, you always want to get the fullest benefits from your workouts as you can. Besides using my 3-F Formula, follow these intensity principles and you'll be on your way to creating a shapely, defined body.

ALTERNATE UPPER- AND LOWER-BODY MOVES

By alternating upper- and lower-body exercises, your body is being constantly challenged in a way that helps burn more calories and more fat—plus keeps your metabolism high. While giving your upper body a rest, you work your lower body, and vice versa. This produces twice the results.

GO HEAVY WITH RESISTANCE

When you do use weights, don't be a wimp. A lot of people make the mistake of using very light weights. They think that more reps will help burn calories and body fat, but in reality this is an ineffective way to train. You've got to use a resistance heavy enough that your muscles are on fire for the last five to eight reps in your set. Muscle tissue burns fat—and the best way to build muscle is by lifting heavier with great form. By adding 5 to 10 percent more resistance to your moves and performing sets in the fifteen- to thirty-rep range, you shock your metabolism to burn even faster. This kind of intensity burns six hundred extra calories in the two days following your workout!

BUST TRAINING PLATEAUS

After one month of working out, you will hit a plateau and discover that no matter what you do you're not getting the results you want. This typically happens if you have been following the same routine for a while, exercising your muscle groups in the same pattern or sequence and not increasing your poundages or repetitions. Muscles get bored and, after some time, their tissues don't regenerate the way they did at the start of your workout phase. One of the best ways of breaking out of a plateau is to jack up the intensity of your workouts. You can do this by increasing your poundages, reps, or changing up your exercises once a month. The same goes for cardio too. You've got to up your speed, duration, and resistance once a month.

KEEP YOUR WORKOUTS SHORT

You don't need two hours in the gym every day to achieve a rock-hard body. The people who spend that much time in the gym are usually athletes or hanging out and socializing. All you need is a thirty-minute resistance training workout, preceded by a twenty-minute interval cardio workout, as I outlined in chapter 8. Stay focused and work intensely. If you're not burning and sweating, then you're not using correct form or enough weight.

SHAKE IT UP

Doing the same thing over and over, hoping for a different result, is called insanity! Change your program so that your body keeps changing. Being stuck and not making progress is known as plateauing, and you want to avoid it at all costs. Fortunately, you have a number of Power Circuits to choose from, right here in this chapter. So after about a month, to keep making progress, switch to another Power Circuit routine and increase your resistance. This will give your body new challenges and compel it to change in the direction of the goals you've set.

REDUCE YOUR REST TIME BETWEEN SETS

The less rest time, the more human growth hormone (HGH) your body releases through exercise. And as I've said, HGH signals the body to build muscle and burn fat. Minimizing rest between sets also pumps more fat-burning oxygen through your system.

Don't Overthink

My trainers always tell their clients: *Don't think about it, just do it.* And guess what? They get results. The concept of *don't think, do* intrigued me, so I decided to research the truth behind it. I learned that successful exercisers really don't think about having to train, they just get out and do it. Sandra Cousins, EdD, an exercise gerontologist at the University of Alberta in Edmonton, has studied this phenomenon herself. She found that people who relied on self pep talks to try to motivate themselves remained couch potatoes, because they actually talked themselves out of exercising! The lesson here: The more you talk about it, the more exhausted and stressed out you might get about it. Find that fire and go!

Evaluate Your Progress Regularly

Keep a training log and have your routine planned out before you start. I always pre-write my routines because it makes me accountable. If I know I'm expected to do my legs routine because it's written out, I'm more likely to follow through. Also, it's an absolute must to track your reps, sets, and increases with resistance training. Over time, your written log will help you identify strengths, weaknesses, and improvements in your physique. Seeing your progress on paper is incredibly motivating. You'll be encouraged and inspired when you look back on your entries and see how far you've come.

In your training log, be sure to note any significant feelings, mental or physical, that occur in response to working out. If I'm not sore after my back routine, for example, I make a note of this. This feedback tells me I need to change weight or exercise groupings. On the other hand, put a smiley face next to the days when working out made you feel sore. Soreness means great things are happening to your muscles. Keeping tabs on your progress (or lack thereof) is the only way to accurately assess your progress, stay accountable, and devise solutions to problems. I still carry my battered little training log to the gym every day. I've provided a sample training log for you in appendix C.

TAKE YOUR MEASUREMENTS

Grab a cloth tape measure and take your before measurements now and your after measurements a month from now. The best areas to measure are:

* Your chest: Across the middle of your breasts. Keep the tape measure level around your body.

* Your waist: Around your belly button.

* Hips: Around the widest part of your hip area.

* Thighs: Around the largest part of both thighs.

* Biceps: Flex and measure around the largest part.

In the chart below, record your weight and measurements.

MY MEASUREMENTS

BEFORE Date:	AFTER Date:
Chest:	Chest:
Waist:	Waist:
Hips:	Hips:
Right Thigh:	Right Thigh:
Left Thigh:	Left Thigh:
Right Biceps:	Right Biceps:
Left Biceps:	Left Biceps:

When taking these measurements, do it at an appropriate time, like in the morning. For example, you wouldn't want to take your waist measurement after you eat a treat meal.

After a month, get the tape measure out again and get excited about your changing shape. You might have lost inches all over. You may have gained inches in a good way. Instead of a flat butt, you may have developed a tighter, higher butt. The overall shape of your body will change with more muscle and less fat. Your clothes should fit differently in one month's time.

And One More Thing . . . Crunches Are a Waste of Time

I came up with this phrase to combat my total frustration at seeing constant ab machine infomercials and prominent trainers peddling ab exercise balls on TV and promising weight loss and a six-pack. Doing hundreds of crunches on any contraption won't help you lose weight. It's a total disservice to the public when professionals sell that concept to you. The only muscles that help you burn fat are the large muscles of the body, such as quadriceps or pectorals. This means that a push-up, because it works your chest, is a better fat burner and core builder. I'm not saying that training your abs isn't important; it's just that many ab exercises like crunches aren't going to make you thinner. Also, if you focus only on crunches, you won't lose weight from your belly, and you may build some muscle under your fat—which will make your waistline larger! So doing endless crunches is a waste of time.

An effective way to trim inches from your midsection, in addition to doing large-muscle core work, is to do two to three ab exercises at the end of your Power Circuit routine. Also, change the combination of those exercises each time to keep those muscles challenged. Another tip to burn ab fat is to contract your abdominal muscles while doing any kind of cardiovascular exercise like Spinning or running. Diet changes such as reducing alcohol consumption or cutting out refined sugar during the week will really burn off belly fat and allow your six-pack to emerge.

My Power Circuit Routines

Okay—it's time to start my fat-burning, boredom-busting, attitude-enhancing program. Look at your calendar and figure out when you can truly allot fifty minutes, three days a week, to this program. Your fifty-minute workout will include a twenty-minute interval cardio and your thirty-minute resistance-training routine.

We all have an optimal strength period in which our body is more energized and stronger. If you know you're too tired after work, for example, don't even try to work out. Schedule a morning time, and keep the appointment. That way, you're setting yourself up for success. You'll feel amazing accomplishment throughout the day by getting it done and doing it at a time compatible with your body's energy level.

Workout Guidelines

1. There are three different Power Circuit routines: routine A, routine B, and routine C. You'll be doing two exercises for each muscle group and alternating between your upper body and lower body, and arms and core.

2. Perform your Power Circuit three times a week. As an example, you can do routine A on Monday; routine B on Wednesday; and routine C on Friday.

3. Perform 1 set of each exercise for 15 to 30 repetitions, then immediately move on to the next exercise with only a few seconds of rest in between. To burn fat, you stay on the move.

4. Begin each routine with the warm-up exercises and finish with the cool-down stretches.

5. After one month, increase your weights. Mix and match your exercises as long as you do two exercises for each muscle group and alternate between your upper and lower body and arms and core.

6. Begin your workout with a warm-up.

The Warm-Up

CHAIN BREAKERS:

15 repetitions

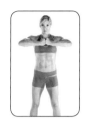 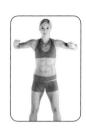

KNEE-UPS:

60 reps, alternating

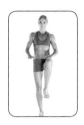 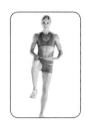

JUMPING JACKS:

60 reps

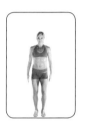 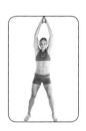

SHOULDER CROSSOVERS:

30 reps

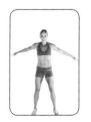 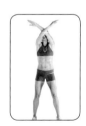

HEAD ROLLS:

15 reps

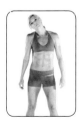 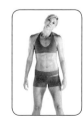

The Routines

Completion of one full routine is the equivalent of one set. Each routine should be performed three times straight through in order of exercises.

Routine A

Choose weights heavy enough so that when performing a set it's difficult to squeeze out the last five reps and still maintain good form. After one month, be sure to change up your routine to prevent a plateau. Increase your poundages, your reps, or both.

CIRCUIT 1

Chest Exercises

DUMBBELL PRESSES WITH TWIST:
15 reps/3 sets

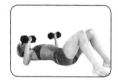 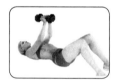

DUMBBELL FLYES:
15 reps/3 sets

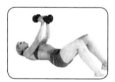 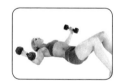

Quadriceps Exercises

UFCs:
30 reps/3 sets/no weight

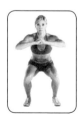 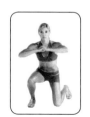 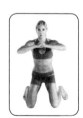 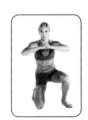

FRONT KICKS:

15 reps each leg/3 sets/
no weight

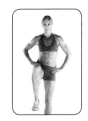
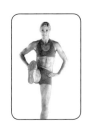

Triceps Exercises

HEADBANGERS:

15 reps/3 sets

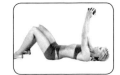
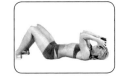

NARROW PRESSES:

15 reps/3 sets

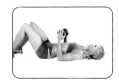

Core Exercises

V-TUCKS:

30 reps/3 sets/no weight

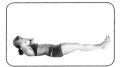

BICYCLE:

30 reps/3 sets/no weight

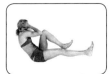
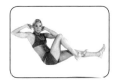

Chest Exercises

DUMBBELL HAMMER PRESSES:
15 reps/3 sets

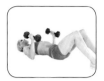 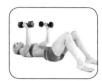 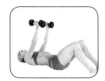

REVERSE DUMBBELL PRESSES:
15 reps/3 sets

 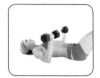

Quadriceps Exercises

SISSY SQUATS:
15 reps each leg/3 sets

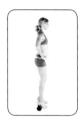 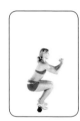

FRONT DUMBBELL LUNGES:
15 reps each leg/3 sets

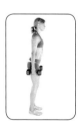 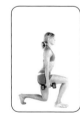

Triceps Exercises

KICKBACKS:

15 reps/3 sets

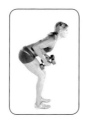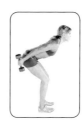

NOSE BUSTERS:

15 reps/3 sets

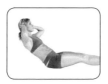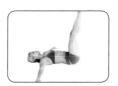

Core Exercises

AB HOLDS:

30 reps/3 sets

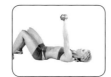

WINDSHIELD WIPERS:

30 reps/3 sets

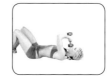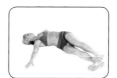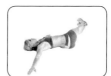

CIRCUIT 3

Chest Exercises

RENEGADE PUSH-UPS:
30 reps/3 sets

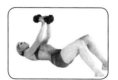 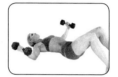 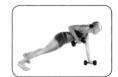

DUMBBELL FLYES:
15 reps/3 sets

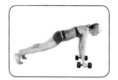 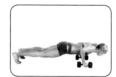

Quadriceps Exercises

UFCs:
30 reps/3 sets

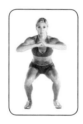 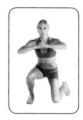 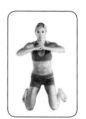 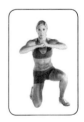

JUMP SQUATS:
15–30 reps/3 sets

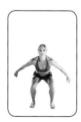 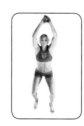

Triceps Exercises

NARROW PRESSES:
15 reps/3 sets

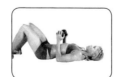

REVERSE POSTERIOR RAISES:

15–30 reps/3 sets

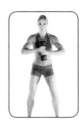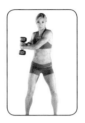

Core Exercises

DUMBBELL TRANSVERSES:

30 reps/3 sets

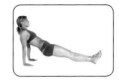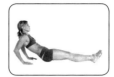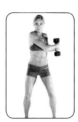

SINGLE-LEG JACKKNIVES:

15 reps each side/3 sets

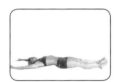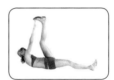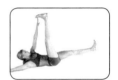

Routine B

Choose weights heavy enough so that when performing a set it's difficult to squeeze out the last five reps and still maintain good form. After one month, be sure to change up your routine to prevent a plateau. Increase your poundages, your reps, or both.

CIRCUIT 1

Back Exercises

WIDE DUMBBELL PULLS:
15 reps/3 sets

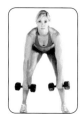 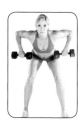

WINGMANS:
30 reps/3 sets

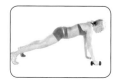 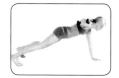

Hamstring Exercises

DUMBBELL DEAD LIFTS:
15 reps/3 sets

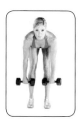 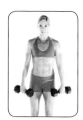

CROSS-KNEE BRIDGES:
15–30 reps/3 sets

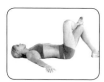 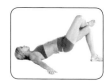

Biceps Exercises

CONCENTRATION CURLS
15 reps/3 sets

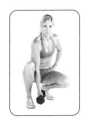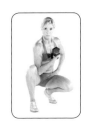

ALTERNATING DUMBBELL CURLS WITH ROTATION:
15 reps/3 sets

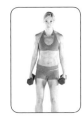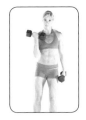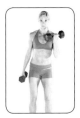

Core Exercises

V-TUCKS:
30 reps/3 sets/no weight

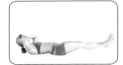

BICYCLE:
30 reps/3 sets/no weight

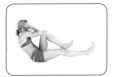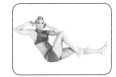

CIRCUIT 2

Back Exercises

ALTERNATING DUMBBELL ROWS:
15 reps/3 sets

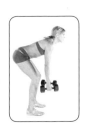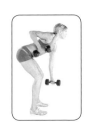

SWIMMERS

30 reps/3 sets

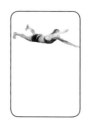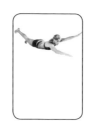

Hamstring Exercises

ALTERNATE SPLIT JUMPS:

30 reps/3 sets

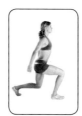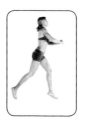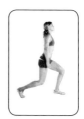

CROSS-KNEE BRIDGES:

15–30 reps/3 sets

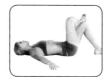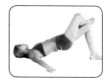

Biceps Exercises

OUTER CURLS:

15 reps/3 sets

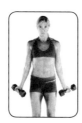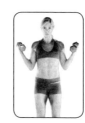

HAMMER CURLS:

15 reps/3 sets

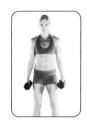 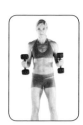

Core Exercises

AB HOLDS:

30 reps/3 sets

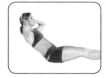

WINDSHIELD WIPERS:

30 reps/3 sets

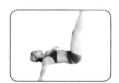 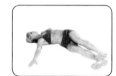 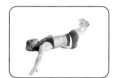

CIRCUIT 3

Back Exercises

WIDE DUMBBELL PULLS:

15 reps/3 sets

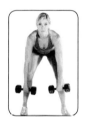 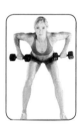

DUMBBELL PULLOVERS:

15 reps/3 sets

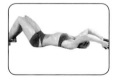 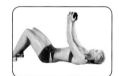

Hamstring Exercises

DUMBBELL DEAD LIFTS:

15 reps/3 sets

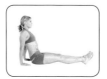 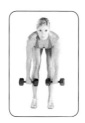 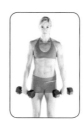 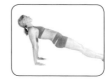

REVERSE PLANKS:

15–30 reps/3 sets

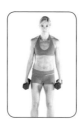 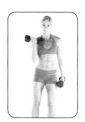

Biceps Exercises

ALTERNATING DUMBBELL CURLS WITH ROTATION:

15 reps/3 sets

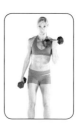

REVERSE CURLS:

15 reps/3 sets

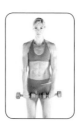 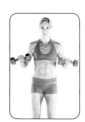

Core Exercises

DUMBBELL TRANSVERSES:
30 reps/3 sets

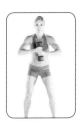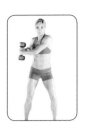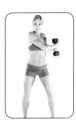

SINGLE-LEG JACKKNIVES:
15 reps each side/3 sets

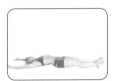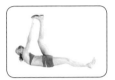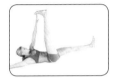

Routine C

Choose weights heavy enough so that when performing a set it's difficult to squeeze out the last five reps and still maintain good form. After one month, be sure to change up your routine to prevent a plateau. Increase your poundages, your reps, or both.

CIRCUIT 1

Glute Exercises

DUMBBELL FRONT SQUATS:
15 reps/3 sets

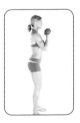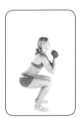

BACK BRIDGES:
15–30 reps/3 sets

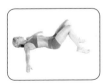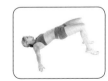

Shoulder Exercises

INS AND OUTS:
15 reps/3 sets

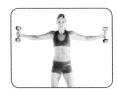

DUMBBELL LATERAL RAISES:
15 reps/3 sets

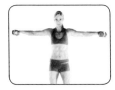

Core Exercises

V-TUCKS:
30 reps/3 sets

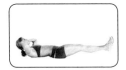

BICYCLE:
30 reps/3 sets

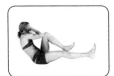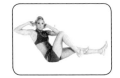

CIRCUIT 2

Glute Exercises

HEISMANS:
30 reps each side/3 sets

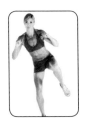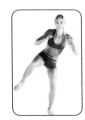

SUMO SQUATS:

15–30 reps/3 sets

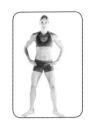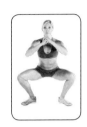

Shoulder Exercises

FRONT RAISES:

15 reps/3 sets

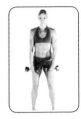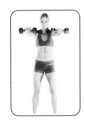

BENTOVER REAR FLYES:

15 reps/3 sets

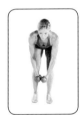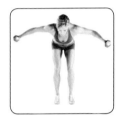

Core Exercises

AB HOLDS:

30 reps/3 sets

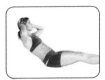

WINDSHIELD WIPERS:

30 reps/3 sets

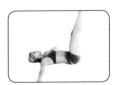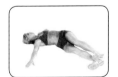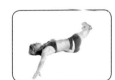

Glute Exercises

DUMBBELL FRONT SQUATS:
15 reps/3 sets

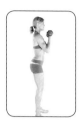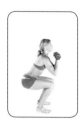

DONKEY-KICK CROSSOVERS:
30 reps/3 sets both legs

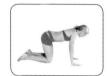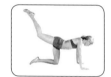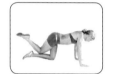

Shoulder Exercises

DUMBBELL LATERAL RAISES:
15 reps/3 sets

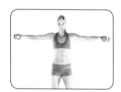

INS AND OUTS:
15 reps/3 sets

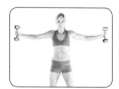

Core Exercises

DUMBBELL TRANSVERSES:
30 reps/3 sets

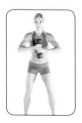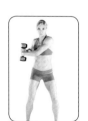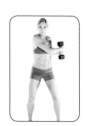

SINGLE-LEG JACKKNIVES:

15 reps each side/3 sets

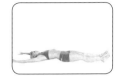 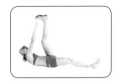 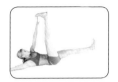

The Cool-Down

HURDLER'S STRETCH:

Hold each stretch 30 seconds.

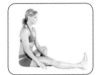 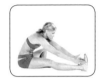

SUMO STRETCH:

Hold each stretch 30 seconds.

KNEE CROSSOVERS:

Hold each stretch 30 seconds.

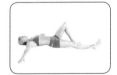 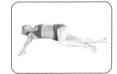

CHEST STRETCH:

Hold each stretch 30 seconds.

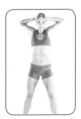

SHOULDER CROSSOVER STRETCH:
Hold each stretch 30 seconds.

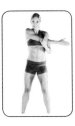

CHILD'S POSE:
Hold each stretch 30 seconds.

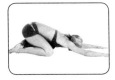

TRICEPS STRETCH:
Hold each stretch 30 seconds.

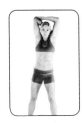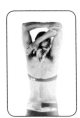

Incorporating Your Cardio

Do your twenty-minute cardio interval work five times a week. Ideally, three of those workouts should be done prior to your resistance-training routine, as I noted above. You can, however, do your cardio apart from the resistance training, on different days or at different times during the day. Regardless of how you organize your workouts, the key is to do five 20-minute interval cardio routines every week.

Muscle Soreness: Love It!

I always tell clients, "If the muscle doesn't burn, it's not working. So make it burn!" The same goes for soreness. If the muscle isn't sore one to two days following your workout, then it's not working. Muscle soreness is a sign of muscle progress. If you're sore after exercising, that's positive. Sore muscles equal toned muscles. That said, if you feel excessively sore following a workout, and you're uncomfortable, do the following:

* Make sure you're supplementing with free-form amino acids daily. They'll help your muscles repair more quickly.

* Mix two tablespoons of baking soda into thirty-two ounces of the water you'll drink daily. Baking soda neutralizes the lactic acid buildup in muscles that causes the soreness.

What to Eat Before and After Exercising

When you eat and what you eat before and after exercising can maximize your results. Here are my guidelines on eating to help better develop your muscles and have more energy for your workouts.

Before Your Workout

If you've had a balanced meal within the last three hours, you shouldn't need to eat anything before hitting the gym. But if it's been longer than three hours since your last meal, or you're working out first thing in the morning, make yourself a protein shake prior to working out. I blend one every morning.

Otherwise, have a light snack about an hour prior to exercising. It should be high in protein. I eat boiled eggs prior to training, for example. Other good pre-workout snacks include nuts, peanut butter on toast, or a cup of oatmeal. Don't grab any sweets or other source of refined sugar, looking for quick energy. Your body won't burn as much fat.

After Your Workout

Consider what happens inside your body as a consequence of intense exercise: Energy-giving glycogen stores are depleted. Muscle protein is dismantled. Microscopic tears in muscle fibers occur, and muscles are inflamed. You never want to "eat" into that fat-burning muscle, so you must supply your body with good nutrition. About an hour after your workout, eat a healthy meal with the right combination of protein, carbs, and fat, like those meals listed in appendix A. If you can't get a full meal in, make sure to have a snack. Some ideal post-workout snacks include:

* Slice of whole-grain or gluten-free bread with turkey breast slices (add desired veggies and mustard)

* Piece of fresh fruit and low-fat cheese

* Handful of raw nuts such as almonds and a piece of fresh fruit

* A whey protein shake blended with half a banana or a cup of fresh berries

* Hummus on whole wheat pita bread

* Tuna drizzled with a little lemon juice and olive oil spread over a slice of whole wheat or gluten-free bread

* Cup of oatmeal

* Grilled chicken and a cup of brown rice

* Low-fat cottage cheese and a piece of fresh fruit

This perfect combo of diet and exercise is going to shock your system in the best way! So get excited and get ready to see real, lasting results.

Part 4

THIS IS HOW YOU STAY HOT AND HEALTHY

11 Metaphysiques

We've talked at length about what causes weight gain—messed-up hormones, too much sugar in your diet, and sluggish organ systems—and what to do about every bit of this. But there's something else working against you—your mind. If you think about being fat, worrying constantly about weight, then you are actively working against yourself! Your negative thoughts and feelings have created your weight problem and have made you unhappy with yourself. It's time for you to break that cycle.

You can do that with "metaphysiques." What is this? Metaphysiques is a powerful mind-body practice I've developed based on using quantum physics to positively influence your body. Without getting too technical about quantum physics, here's how it works: Know that everything in the universe is made up of energy, including your thoughts and feelings, and that "like attracts like." This means your thoughts and feelings are energy that attracts similar energy. So basically, as you think, so you attract.

What does this have to do with weight loss? Everything!

> **In This Chapter:**
>
> * Get thin by thinking thin
> * Attracting health and fitness
> * Move in the direction of your goals
> * Visualize your perfect body into being
> * Take action to have what you really want
> * The pleasure principle

Instead of focusing on being fat, you've got to focus on being fit. If you think healthy, it eventually becomes reality for you. I always push my clients to focus on how strong they're getting, how well they're sleeping, and how happy they're feeling. Choosing to focus on thoughts that feel good, and are positive, is a sure way to create the body you want. The by-product is a beautiful, sexy body. Start thinking exactly how the people with hot, buffed bodies think! They see themselves as attractive, energetic, athletic, and in sync with their bodies. They draw to themselves the best of everything with their thoughts.

At the same time, do not hope, but assume you will lose weight. As in life, great things come to those who work for a goal and assume the outcome will be in their favor. All of these new thoughts and actions will create the thin thighs, the flat stomach, and the hot body you want. You'll be sending out the right energy, and it's energy that creates your new reality.

Long before I developed metaphysiques, I knew I had its power. A power that I practiced. I could change the way people acted around me. I could change the outcome of certain events. I could achieve anything I put my mind to. I understood at a very basic level that my thoughts—and the energy that emanated from those thoughts—could move mountains or start fires. I simply had to choose which to do.

Every one of you has that same power. You can do things you never thought you could do. You will create the body you want, starting with your personal dialogue about yourself. Thoughts and feelings turn into actions, and actions into reality. Remember, you are opening a new chapter in your life, one that is much more in control and energized. Let me show you how to change your life.

Think Thin, Be Thin

A lot of people I know want a better life, more money, a sexy body, or more power over their circumstances. But they don't know how to get there. Why? Because their heads are filled with negative self-talk like *fat, ugly,* or *failure*. This inner self-loathing conversation is toxic and success-blocking. If you're negative about yourself, you'll attract failure. Example: If you think that you *can't* ever lose weight, then you know what? You're right. You won't. The word *can't* gets so stuck in your subconscious mind that your body believes and obeys it! You've trained your mind to believe you can't, and now you've hit a roadblock to success. I don't ever allow clients to say *can't* or *try*. Don't try, do!

Thoughts release neuropeptides—chemicals of emotion—that travel to cells whenever we think or speak. They affect the tension in your muscles, the rate of your heart, your ability to digest your food, your overall health, and more. Angry, bitter, or critical thoughts produce chemicals that depress your immune system, make you sick, and keep you fat. Thinking about something repetitively even alters cell assemblies—collections of brain cells that work together. We use cell assemblies to learn and remember things; they also drive goal-directed behavior. Negative thoughts, often a result of stress, can cause cell assemblies to work in a disorganized manner. We can't recall things as well, and our thinking gets muddled, when we're stressed out.

Thoughts are powerful and vital in creating the energy we put forth, including healing energy. Several years ago, my mother was diagnosed with lymphoma, a cancer of the lymphatic system. In addition to standard therapies, she decided to have Reiki treatment. Reiki is a healing system based on the idea that an unseen *life force energy* flows through us and is what causes us to be alive. This life force is responsive to thoughts and feelings.

The Reiki healer came to my mom's house. She asked my mother to sit in a chair in front of a large window that just happened to be filled with about twenty houseplants. As part of the therapy, the healer imagined a blue, healing light into my mother's body. The purpose of the light was to direct the bad energy out of Mom's body and out the window. And so that's how the therapy went, day after day. What happened within a few weeks was very interesting. Within a month, all the plants in that window died—and my mother went into remission. Healing happens when negative thoughts are exorcised.

I'm not saying you have to do Reiki to get thin or healthy. I'm saying thoughts have power, and you've got to harness that power by changing how you think. If you're getting the same negative results in your life—like weight gain—then you've been consciously or unconsciously running negative tapes through your mind like:

> *I'm a fat pig, and no one is gonna want me.*
> *It's hard to lose weight.*
> *I'll never have a body I want.*

That's negative energy, and I guarantee it will repel positivity. Let's face it: Life can be hell if you are walking around hating your body and being fat. How many times in your life have you said, "I hate my thighs! My butt's too big! My tummy is fat!"? Watch it. Hating any body part makes it fatter. That's the conclusion of a study I read years ago, and I have never forgotten it. Scary, isn't it? Our thoughts can work powerfully for us, or against us. What we focus on expands. Hate your thighs, butt, and abs? Just watch them expand.

How do you get rid of this negativity? First, you have to make yourself aware of it. Much of the dialogue that goes on is so comfortable to us that we don't know it's happening. Second, try to catch yourself thinking negatively about yourself; then say your name out loud followed by *stop*. Third, rephrase your thinking—out loud—to be positive. For example, sometimes I might feel insecure about a photo shoot. A negative inner dialogue starts in my head. To combat those negative thoughts, I say out loud: "Jackie, *stop*. You did your best at that photo shoot and the pictures are going to be beautiful."

See how this works? It's like flipping a switch from a negative, insecure thought to a positive, empowering one. The more you practice this technique, the more your thoughts will change to positive ones automatically, and you won't even have to use the technique anymore.

I also frequently say to myself: *I'm on my way to changing my life and I'm proud that I'm motivated to change*. I push negative thoughts away and instantly replace them with thoughts that are positive. You can do this yourself by coming up with upbeat mantras and repeating them often. For example:

> *I am getting healthier and more beautiful every day.*
> *I love myself and deserve a healthy body.*
> *I don't need fat anymore. I am strong.*
> *Changing my body will change my life.*

Do something else: Use powerful, present-tense verbs to boost yourself to a new thought level. Eliminate weak phrases like, *I'm trying to lose weight . . . I'm planning to exercise . . . I'm hoping to eat healthier*. You're not trying, planning, or hoping! You're doing it. Say so—and you'll subconsciously reinforce success.

Even body language counts. Before my clients even pick up a weight, I have them walk toward themselves in the mirror. I show them that just by looking forward, with their chest out and shoulders back, they actually look ten pounds lighter. Always carry yourself like you mean business and the world will take notice.

Thoughts and feelings have power; they can help or hurt you. Lose the negative thinking and negative emotions and you'll lose the fat.

FAT-BURNING FACT: POSITIVE THINKING SHEDS POUNDS

THINKING POSITIVELY WILL definitely help you shed weight, according to a Harvard study. Scientists found that simply believing that you're doing enough exercise can shed pounds. They made this discovery by monitoring a group of eighty-four female hotel housekeepers who complained that they were not getting any exercise, despite their strenuous jobs. Half of the test subjects were told not to worry and that their work provided them with enough exercise to lose weight and maintain a healthy lifestyle. They were even told how many calories they were burning doing specific tasks such as vacuuming, changing linens, and sweeping floors. The other half were told nothing about the health benefits of their daily chores. All the subjects cleaned about fifteen rooms a day, taking twenty to thirty minutes for each.

After four weeks, the informed group had lost an average of two pounds, lowered their blood pressure by almost 10 percent, and reduced their body fat. The other group had no noticeable changes in health or physique. This study shows that if you can put your mind in a healthy, positive place, believing that you are burning calories or losing weight, you can achieve amazing physiological benefits.

Source: Psychological Science

Goals: Discover What You Really Want

It's really important to stop being wishy-washy about getting thin. Get specific about your fat-loss goals. You can't hit a target you can't see. You can't go through life without goals and expect to get anywhere. You need direction.

Suppose you set out in a strange city to find a specific address, and you're smart enough to have a GPS system. You'll be able to move faster and more dependably from wherever you are to wherever you want to go. Well, you need a GPS system to get thin, too. Goals are your GPS.

Decide on your goals and write them down. The act of writing is visual—it helps you clearly envision each goal—and it's kinesthetic, because you're using your hand, wrist, and arm to write. Visual and kinesthetic actions program those goals into your subconscious mind. The process is like saving it to your hard drive. It becomes a permanent part of your mental operating system, moving you in the direction of your goals—and in time you'll achieve them. When you have conscious goals for a thin, hot body, you'll consciously choose to do anything that supports that intent, like eating better and exercising more.

Make sure your goals are realistic. Instead of saying, "I want to be thin by summer," set goals you can realistically attain. I have noticed that when clients set goals that are athletic- and performance-based, meaning the goals are quantifiable, they are more likely to succeed. For example:

* Jog six times around your block four times a week.

* Eat clean for five days in a row.

* Increase your weight resistance by five to ten pounds in one month.

* Compete in one mini marathon this year.

When you write down your goals, your conscious mind will desire those goals, but your unconscious fears of failure and loss may cause you to doubt yourself. The solution is to make a list of every single thing that you could do to achieve the goal. When

> ## THE POWER OF THE PLACEBO EFFECT
>
> EVER HEARD OF the placebo effect? A placebo, or sugar pill, is a substance that, by itself, has no effect on the body. But when a placebo is combined with the power of suggestion, almost anything is possible. It means if you believe a treatment works, you'll feel better, or possibly be cured. People who expect positive results from medical treatments are more likely to get them. All this is called the placebo effect. It's proof that our thoughts, feelings, and attitudes can push us toward illness or health.

you do this, something happens to your doubts: They begin to dissipate. Simultaneously, your confidence and faith in the attainment of those goals increase.

So write down your own goals, and the steps you'll take to achieve them. With each step toward your goal, you become more confident. At a certain point, you move from "positive thinking" to "positive knowing." You absolutely know, deep inside, that you will attain your goals.

Visualize

Train your mind to achieve your goals with visualization. I call this "motivational day-dreaming." Athletes do it all the time. A basketball player might visualize swishing a last-second jump shot, or a baseball player might visualize hitting a home run.

Personally, I have practiced visualization since I was a child. For example, I always knew I would someday speak in front of a large audience, because I fantasized about it for years. And guess what? Bravo gave me a TV show.

As a young adult, I had a recurring dream that I was living in a penthouse apartment overlooking the city at night. I assumed this meant that I would be rich someday, living in a luxurious penthouse suite—haha. Fast-forward twenty years: After being cheated out of my first gym business, I was desperately searching for office space to start a new gym. My Realtor was showing me space on the sixth floor of a medical building and asked if I wanted to see the view from up top. The elevator doors opened and there I was in the penthouse at night overlooking the city. I felt as if someone had grabbed my heart. My dream had been about SkySport, my gym. I knew this was a sign and I moved mountains, selling everything I had to make that dream a reality. SkySport brought me my TV show, and a wonderful career and life. The power of the unconscious mind, combined with hard work, turns dream into reality. Speaking positively to yourself will change your unconscious feelings about yourself, which will change what the universe brings you.

I'm sure you've also heard about patients using visualization to help heal their diseases—a broken bone being knit back together, for example, or a tumor shrinking down to nothing. These images work their way into the nervous system, the immune system, the organs, muscles, bones, and other tissues to enable healing. In a study conducted by researchers from the University of Texas School of Public Health and M. D. Anderson Cancer

Center, forty-seven women who had just undergone treatment for breast cancer participated in six-week sessions of a support group and guided imagery (where they learned to imagine their immune cells overtaking cancer cells, for example). The results of the study suggested that the therapies boosted immune function in the women who participated in the imagery and support groups. The study was published in *Alternative Therapies in Health and Medicine.* Thinking yourself well is a very powerful force for healing.

Visualize with your conscious mind and your thoughts will start to pervade your unconscious mind. When both the conscious and unconscious minds are shifted toward the positive, you will be unstoppable. You can use these powerful forces for weight loss, because you are what you think. To help yourself lose weight, see yourself getting healthier. Focus on health and a smaller size will come. That's because the body doesn't know the difference between what's really happening and what your mind is telling it. To your mind, it's as if you already have a great body. This internal image controls what you focus on, what you attract, and what you do. If you see yourself as a thin, hot, sexy person, then you'll do things—like eating right and working out—in line with that image.

So dream it into being, like a movie in your head, and be detailed:

* Envision yourself at your dream weight, in a bikini, having child-like fun with friends by the pool.

* Visualize yourself confidently flirting or finding your inner sexiness with someone.

* Picture yourself in great shape, jogging on the beach in Rio.

* Imagine yourself exercising and loving it. This strengthens the mental connection between exercise and you. See yourself going through a whole set without getting tired, and feel the power flowing through your muscles. As you do this, think of positive words, such as *strong, confident,* and *energetic.* When you're actually doing your workout, you'll reexperience those feelings of confidence and strength.

Do your visualizations when you wake up in the morning, before you go to bed at night, or when you're exercising. Workouts are life-enhancing meditation. My best, purest

> ## TRICKS OF THE TRADE: SEE YOURSELF AS AN ATHLETE
>
> **AN IMPORTANT PART** of metaphysiques is whether or not you see yourself as an athlete, or at least a physically active person. When I tell my clients that I see the athlete in them, they actually work harder and complete those last five reps. Your behavior is consistent with your identity. In other words, the way you see yourself determines your actions and behavior. Therefore, with regard to exercise, the more you identify with physical activity as part of who you are, the more likely you are to stick to physical activity and make it part of your lifestyle.
>
> I challenge you to take a good, hard look at how you see yourself. When you look in the mirror, do you see a lazy, fat, out-of-shape person? If so, your behavior will follow to match that identity—you will in effect act like and be a lazy, fat, out-of-shape person. You'll hesitate to put on your gym clothes, because you'll be saying to yourself, *What am I thinking? I'm no exerciser! Just look at all this ugly flesh!*
>
> On the other hand, if you see your inner athlete, motivated to change . . . guess what? You become that person. It's your choice.

ideas of what I want to achieve have come when I'm in the middle of training. Your workout is your positive connection to your body, energy, and mind.

Voice your goals and passions with as many people as possible. The more you talk about them, the more you imprint and program them into your subconscious mind. Talking the talk will lead to walking the walk.

Believe you already have the body of your dreams. You don't have to have proof that you will get there. You simply need to believe it, and you'll automatically take the right actions to get there.

Visualize, visualize, visualize—then be prepared to be amazed at how good you start to feel. You'll be even more amazed by the results. Work on your head, and your body will follow.

Act to Get What You Want

Metaphysiques is more than simply wishing for what you want. You can't sit around like a magnet, waiting to attract the things you want. Most people underachieve or fail because they never get going in the first place. And if they do get going, they allow themselves to slow down and stop, making it almost impossible for them to energize again. Don't let this happen to you.

Keep this in mind: The last six letters in *attraction* are *action*. Successful people are intensely action-oriented. They move in the direction of their desires.

Action works best when surrounded by all of the other things I talked about above: changing your thoughts, setting goals, visualizing them daily, and affirming that you have that which you are working toward. Metaphysiques essentially means: Be, Do, Have. The "be" is being a positive person, with empowering thoughts, beliefs, and feelings. The "do" is visualizing, setting goals, and acting. The "have" is the outcome of being and doing. There is a connection among all three, and one without the other will stall your progress.

The "doing" part of metaphysiques also involves eating right and exercising hard. But you don't have to force yourself to do this. You'll do it with happiness and ease because you see yourself that way, guided by your desires, goals, and visualizations.

The actions of good nutrition and exercise create even more positive energy that you project to the world. You see, the foods you eat have a huge effect on how

> ### GET HOT AND HEALTHY, BE SUCCESSFUL
>
> **LIKE IT OR NOT,** people judge you on how you look, and that extends to the workplace. According to a survey published in *Personnel Today,* an astonishing 93 percent of human resource professionals said they would hire a "normal weight" candidate rather than an overweight person who was identically qualified. Lots of other polls have come up with similar findings. Okay, so this isn't fair. But this is the world we live in.
>
> Lose weight, pay attention to the details of your appearance, and you'll project a confident business image. Other amazing things will follow. It's foolish not to use your body and looks to your advantage and make the most with what you've got. Appearance counts for a lot in the job world. If you don't think so, you're naive or possibly out of a job.

you feel mentally. When you put clean, energy-giving foods into your system, and exercise with intensity, your body produces positive body chemicals. These chemicals enable both the body and the mind to break free of rigid, negative patterns. They promote feelings of accomplishment and control and help break the vicious cycle of sluggishness and depression. They allow you to radiate high energy that attracts into your world anything you want—the ability to get thin, build self-esteem and self-respect, achieve success—anything.

I have used fitness, nutrition, and metaphysiques to change my energy and change my own life. Everything positive that has happened to me in my adult life is related to nutrition and exercise. I have achieved amazing things like fame, wealth, and love when regularly working out and eating well. Why? Energy! My energy and the way I carry myself in the world completely change because nutrition and exercise make powerful chemicals of well-being course through my system. Every interaction at work, on the streets, and in personal relationships is electric. So give your body what it needs and wants—and watch your weight change and watch your life change.

THE PLEASURE LINKS

USE THESE AFFIRMATIONS and techniques to link nutrition and exercise to pleasure:

* Clean, energy-giving foods help your system produce positive chemicals and work properly to take care of you all day.

* Workouts pump feel-good chemicals throughout your system, and change your self-esteem and your shape. The one hour you put into your body is immediate— but lasts all day. Your metabolism goes up that same hour, and your brain starts associating that energy as very positive.

* Think of the endorphin/dopamine high you get after exercising, or the physical and mental energy you feel after a clean week of eating, instead of holding on to the feelings of failure from inaction or falling off the wagon.

* Listen to your favorite music while working out. This will help you link your workout to pleasure; plus, music drives you to push yourself and inspires movement.

I can say this with conviction, too, because I've helped many people succeed over their weight challenges by changing the way they think and the way they act. Once my clients start applying metaphysiques, I see a newfound energy in them and on their faces. They're eating and exercising because they *want* to do it, because they have now become passionate about themselves. When that happens, it's not *effort*. They've set into motion a whole new life.

Instead of wasting time being angry or depressed that things aren't going well, switch to a positive attitude and positive action and things will get better. If losing weight is a constant goal, step up to the plate and do something about it. Stop the excuses—which lead to more disappointments—and get things done.

Use the Pleasure Principle

Many years ago, I listened to motivational speaker Tony Robbins. He was very inspirational and taught metaphysical principles way before they were popular. I started using one of his principles and applied it to diet and exercise. It's called the Pleasure Principle. Basically, he said that you should link everything in life to pleasure or pain because we are highly motivated by both. Most people think of a diet as miserable deprivation and avoid embarking on that painful journey. What if you looked at a diet as an exciting start to a new life? A way to nourish your body and make it beautiful? Most people look at a plate of cupcakes and think, *Pleasure, pleasure, pleasure.* I don't. I look at them and visualize myself getting photographed in next to nothing and having feelings of insecurity. Yes, I work hard for this body, but I still have insecurities! So, unless it's during a treat meal, I see junk food as causing great pain. Literally attach visions and feelings of pain or pleasure to everything. You will find that many of the things you once linked to pleasure (eating junk food or frequent drinking nights) are actually causing you a tremendous amount of pain, and the things you used to link to pain (workouts or eating healthy) will ultimately give you the greatest rewards.

You have powers you never dreamed of. And now you have all the tools to tap into them. What you are thinking, feeling, and doing now is creating your new life. Your confident mind and your strong body will open unimaginable doors. You are in control of what may happen today and tomorrow. Stop wishing that you had a hot, sexy body and fantastic life and start creating them!

Allow yourself to think about the good for yourself and tell yourself that you deserve to get what you want. Don't settle for less. Celebrate who you are becoming and get excited for this new adventure. You have the power over your body and your life, so live it with passion.

Appendix A

> *Hot and Healthy Meal Plans and Recipes*

Here are sample menus that show you exactly how to eat. The first five days feature menus that incorporate recipes that you'll find here. The rest of the menus (31 days' worth) feature meals for those of you who don't want to prepare recipes. By choosing a variety of foods from my food lists, you'll easily get your complement of hormone balancers and detox foods. Each main meal equals approximately 400 calories; snacks equal around 100 to 150 calories. The menus contain the correct daily allotment of four proteins, three veggies, two fruits, two grains, and one fat.

Menus If You Love to Cook

(The recipes begin on page 237.)

Day 1

BREAKFAST

Goat Cheese and Tomato Basil Omelet (page 242)

Choice of: 1 orange, ½ grapefruit, 1 cup chopped mango, 2 kiwi fruits, or other fresh fruit

MIDMORNING SNACK

2 tablespoons almond or peanut butter on 6 whole-grain crackers

LUNCH

Asian Turkey Lettuce Wraps (page 252)

1 piece fresh fruit, any type

MIDAFTERNOON SNACK

Grilled Stuffed Zucchini Rolls (page 279)

DINNER

Cherry Tomato Salmon (page 262)

1 cup cooked brown rice

1 cup steamed vegetables, any type

POSTDINNER

1 cup decaf green tea mixed with a favorite herbal tea

Day 2

BREAKFAST

1 cup Greek-style yogurt

1 banana

1 slice whole-grain toast with 1 pat butter

MIDMORNING SNACK

1 cup chopped fresh fruit, any type

LUNCH

Grilled Vegetable Chicken Bowl (page 254)

MIDAFTERNOON SNACK

Caprese Kebab (page 276)

DINNER

Thai Beef Stir-Fry (page 259)

1 cup cooked brown rice

POSTDINNER

1 cup decaf green tea mixed with a favorite herbal tea

Day 3

BREAKFAST

Oatmeal, 1 cup

¼ melon

MIDMORNING SNACK

1 pear

1 ounce low-fat cheddar cheese

LUNCH

Pizza Margarita (page 280)

Tossed salad with 1 tablespoon salad dressing

MIDAFTERNOON SNACK

Deviled Tomatoes (page 278)

DINNER

Spicy Herb Chicken (page 266)

1 cup steamed vegetables: broccoli or spinach

POSTDINNER

1 cup decaf green tea mixed with a favorite herbal tea

Day 4

BREAKFAST

Burrito Italiano (page 241)

MIDMORNING SNACK

1 cup chopped pineapple

1 tablespoon raw almonds

LUNCH

1 cup lentil or bean soup

Tossed Caesar salad (romaine lettuce) with 1 tablespoon low-fat
Caesar salad dressing

MIDAFTERNOON SNACK

Whey protein shake blended with 1 cup fresh strawberries

DINNER

4 ounces lean hamburger patty, grilled or broiled

1 cup stewed tomatoes

1 cup cooked brown rice

POSTDINNER

1 cup decaf green tea mixed with a favorite herbal tea

Day 5

BREAKFAST

1 cup oatmeal with 2 tablespoons walnuts or sunflower seeds sprinkled on top,
sweetened with cinnamon and Truvia (stevia-based sweetener)

1 piece fresh fruit, any type

MIDMORNING SNACK

Whey protein shake

LUNCH

Tuna salad on lettuce and sliced tomato: water-packed tuna mixed
with ¼ cup chopped celery, 2 tablespoons chopped onion,
and 1 tablespoon low-fat mayonnaise

1 cup fresh blueberries

MIDAFTERNOON SNACK

2 boiled eggs

DINNER

Steak Fajitas (page 267)

Mexican Rice (page 272)

POSTDINNER

1 cup decaf green tea mixed with a favorite herbal tea

Menus If You're a Noncooker Like Me!

(Day 1)————————————————————————————

BREAKFAST

2 low-fat whole wheat tortillas, each filled with 1 scrambled egg
and 1 tablespoon salsa

MIDMORNING SNACK

1 cup low-fat cottage cheese

1 piece fresh fruit

LUNCH

Mixed veggie salad with chicken breast and 2 tablespoons salad dressing

1 slice whole-grain bread

MIDAFTERNOON SNACK

1 banana

DINNER

4 ounces pork tenderloin

1 cup steamed veggies

1 baked yam

POSTDINNER

1 cup decaf green tea mixed with a favorite herbal tea

(Day 2)————————————————————————

BREAKFAST

Whey protein shake blended with a handful of fresh spinach

1 cup frozen mixed berries

MIDMORNING SNACK

1 cup oatmeal with 2 tablespoons walnuts or sunflower seeds sprinkled on top, sweetened with cinnamon and Truvia (stevia-based sweetener)

LUNCH

2 cans (3 ounces each for a total of 6 ounces) water-packed tuna mixed with 1 tablespoon low-fat mayonnaise on a generous bed of greens

6 whole-grain crackers

MIDAFTERNOON SNACK

2 boiled eggs

DINNER

4 ounces grilled chicken with 1 cup asparagus or mixed veggies

1 cup chopped fresh pineapple

POSTDINNER

1 cup decaf green tea mixed with a favorite herbal tea

Day 3

BREAKFAST

Whey protein shake, 1 serving, blended with 1 cup fresh berries

Oatmeal, 1 cup

MIDMORNING SNACK

2 tablespoons almonds

LUNCH

Dark green leafy salad with salad vegetables (green peppers, cucumbers, onions, et cetera) with 1 tablespoon low-fat salad dressing and 4 ounces grilled chicken breast

Whole-grain bread, 1 slice

MIDAFTERNOON SNACK

1 apple

Low-fat mozzarella cheese, 1 stick

DINNER

4 ounces grilled sirloin steak

1 cup steamed broccoli

1 sweet potato, baked

POSTDINNER

1 cup decaf green tea mixed with a favorite herbal tea

Day 4

BREAKFAST

2 poached eggs

1 slice whole-grain toast with 1 pat butter

Choice of: 1 orange, ½ grapefruit, 1 cup chopped mango, or 2 kiwi fruits

MIDMORNING SNACK

1 cup low-fat cottage cheese

LUNCH

Pita sandwich: 1 whole-grain pita, 2 ounces low-fat feta cheese, 1 cup alfalfa
sprouts, 1 small tomato (sliced), 1 tablespoon olive oil & vinegar dressing

MIDAFTERNOON SNACK

1 apple or other fruit in season

DINNER

4 ounces broiled or grilled sirloin steak

1 medium sweet potato

1 cup steamed veggies, such as yellow wax beans and carrots

POSTDINNER

1 cup decaf green tea mixed with a favorite herbal tea

 Day 5

BREAKFAST

1 cup low-fat cottage cheese

1 slice whole-grain toast with 1 pat butter

½ grapefruit

MIDMORNING SNACK

Whey protein shake

LUNCH

Shrimp salad: large bed of green leafy vegetables and sliced tomato,
topped with 4 ounces boiled shrimp and 1 tablespoon olive oil
& balsamic vinegar dressing

MIDAFTERNOON SNACK

1 large peach, sliced

DINNER

4 ounces roast Cornish game hen, skin removed

1 cup winter squash

POSTDINNER

1 cup decaf green tea mixed with a favorite herbal tea

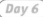 *Day 6* ————————————————————————————————————

BREAKFAST

1 cup Greek-style yogurt

1 cup oatmeal

MIDMORNING SNACK

Whey protein shake blended with one cup sliced strawberries

LUNCH

Greek pocket sandwich: ¼ cup reduced-fat feta cheese mixed with 1 tablespoon vinaigrette salad dressing, ½ cup chopped romaine lettuce, 2 tablespoons each minced onion, celery, and grated carrot, all put into whole wheat pita bread

MIDAFTERNOON SNACK

1 banana

DINNER

4 ounces grilled steak

1 cup butternut squash

1 cup steamed green beans, broccoli, zucchini, or cauliflower

POSTDINNER

1 cup decaf green tea mixed with a favorite herbal tea

(**Day 7**)

BREAKFAST

2 boiled eggs

1 cup corn grits with a pat of butter

1 nectarine

MIDMORNING SNACK

Yogurt parfait: (1 cup Greek-style yogurt, layered with sliced banana)

LUNCH

4 ounces grilled chicken breast

3 new potatoes, boiled

1 cup steamed green beans

MIDAFTERNOON SNACK

½ avocado, sliced, and 1 cup chopped assorted veggies

DINNER

4 ounces grilled steak

2-bean salad: ½ cup kidney beans and 1 cup yellow wax beans
   on a generous bed of lettuce, drizzled with 2 teaspoons olive oil
   & 2 tablespoons balsamic vinegar

1 cup steamed asparagus

POSTDINNER

1 cup decaf green tea mixed with a favorite herbal tea

(**Day 8**)

BREAKFAST

2 scrambled eggs

1 cup cooked cornmeal

½ grapefruit

MIDMORNING SNACK

2 tablespoons raw almond butter with 3 celery sticks

LUNCH

4 ounces baked chicken breast

1 cup steamed summer squash

MIDAFTERNOON SNACK

1 cup chopped mango or other tropical fruit

DINNER

4 ounces grilled sirloin steak

1 cup combined brown and wild rice

1 cup steamed broccoli or cauliflower

POSTDINNER

1 cup decaf green tea mixed with a favorite herbal tea

(**Day 9**)

BREAKFAST

2 low-fat whole wheat tortillas; each filled with 1 scrambled egg
and 1 tablespoon salsa

2 clementines

MIDMORNING SNACK

1 ounce any low-calorie cheese with 1 cup chopped raw veggies
(carrots, green peppers, cucumbers, etc.)

LUNCH

Mixed veggie salad (lettuce, tomatoes, bell peppers, onions—virtually
any salad vegetable), topped with 4 ounces grilled chicken breast
and 2 tablespoons salad dressing

1 slice Ezekiel bread or any dark, nutty bread

MIDAFTERNOON SNACK

1 banana and 10 nuts (such as almonds or walnuts)

DINNER

4 ounces grilled or baked white fish such as tilapia or orange roughy

1 cup steamed yellow wax beans

1 baked yam

POSTDINNER

1 cup decaf green tea mixed with a favorite herbal tea

(Day 10)

BREAKFAST

Whey protein shake blended with 1 handful frozen spinach and 1 cup frozen strawberries

MIDMORNING SNACK

1 cup oat bran with 2 tablespoons walnuts or sunflower seeds sprinkled on top, sweetened with cinnamon and Truvia (stevia-based sweetener)

LUNCH

4 ounces steamed shrimp (chopped), mixed with 1 tablespoon low-fat mayonnaise and served on a generous bed of greens

6 whole-grain crackers

MIDAFTERNOON SNACK

2 boiled eggs

DINNER

4 ounces baked turkey breast

1 cup steamed asparagus

1 cup chopped fresh melon (such as watermelon or cantaloupe)

POSTDINNER

1 cup decaf green tea mixed with a favorite herbal tea

Day 11

BREAKFAST

Whey protein shake blended with 1 cup frozen blueberries

1 cup oatmeal

MIDMORNING SNACK

2 tablespoons almonds

1 apple

LUNCH

Salmon salad: dark green leafy salad with salad vegetables (lettuce, green peppers, cucumbers, onions, etc.), plus chilled steamed green beans with 1 tablespoon low-fat salad dressing and 4 ounces grilled or baked salmon

1 slice whole-grain bread

MIDAFTERNOON SNACK

1 cup beans (kidney beans, black beans, garbanzo beans, etc.)

Low-fat mozzarella cheese, 1 stick

DINNER

4 ounces baked pork tenderloin

1 cup greens (spinach, mustard greens, etc.)

1 baked sweet potato

POSTDINNER

1 cup decaf green tea mixed with a favorite herbal tea

(*Day 12*)

BREAKFAST

2 poached eggs

1 slice whole-grain toast, with 1 pat butter

Choice of: 1 orange, ½ grapefruit, 1 cup chopped mango, or 2 kiwi fruits

MIDMORNING SNACK

1 cup low-fat cottage cheese

LUNCH

Pita sandwich: 1 whole-grain pita pocket, 2 ounces low-fat feta cheese,
1 cup alfalfa sprouts, 1 small tomato (sliced), 1 tablespoon olive oil
& vinegar dressing

MIDAFTERNOON SNACK

1 apple with 2 tablespoons raw almond butter

DINNER

4 ounces broiled or grilled chicken breast

1 medium sweet potato

1 cup steamed zucchini

POSTDINNER

1 cup decaf green tea mixed with a favorite herbal tea

(*Day 13*)

BREAKFAST

1 cup low-fat cottage cheese

1 slice whole-grain toast with 1 pat butter

½ grapefruit

MIDMORNING SNACK

Whey protein shake with 1 cup frozen raspberries

LUNCH

Shrimp or chicken salad: large bed of green leafy vegetables and sliced tomato, topped with 4 ounces boiled shrimp or chicken and 1 tablespoon dressing of olive oil & balsamic vinegar

1 piece of Ezekiel bread or dark, nutty bread

MIDAFTERNOON SNACK

1 large peach with 1 ounce low-calorie cheese

DINNER

4 ounces roast turkey, skin removed

1 cup winter squash

1 cup brown rice

POSTDINNER

1 cup decaf green tea mixed with a favorite herbal tea

(Day 14)

BREAKFAST

1 cup Greek-style yogurt

1 orange

1 slice whole-grain toast with 1 pat butter

MIDMORNING SNACK

1 cup chopped fresh fruit, any type

10 nuts (such as almonds or walnuts)

LUNCH

Grilled vegetables (zucchini or summer squash, onions, bell peppers, etc.)

4 ounces breast of chicken or turkey

MIDAFTERNOON SNACK

2 tablespoons almond or peanut butter on 6 whole-grain crackers

DINNER

Filet mignon (size of your palm)

1 cup cooked brown rice

Large tossed salad with 1 tablespoon fat-free salad dressing

POSTDINNER

1 cup decaf green tea mixed with a favorite herbal tea

(Day 15)

BREAKFAST

1 cup oatmeal

1 cup fresh cherries or other fruit in season

MIDMORNING SNACK

1 pear

1 ounce low-fat cheddar cheese

LUNCH

1 cup beans (kidney beans, black beans, garbanzo beans, etc.)

Large tossed salad with 1 tablespoon salad dressing

MIDAFTERNOON SNACK

2 boiled eggs

DINNER

1 baked Cornish hen, skin removed

1 cup steamed broccoli or spinach

1 cup combined brown and wild rice

POSTDINNER

1 cup decaf green tea mixed with a favorite herbal tea

(Day 16)

BREAKFAST

1 cup oatmeal with cinnamon and Truvia

1 cup blueberries

MIDMORNING SNACK

1 cup chopped fresh pineapple

1 tablespoon raw almonds

LUNCH

1 cup vegetarian lentil or bean soup

Tossed Caesar salad (romaine lettuce) with 1 tablespoon low-fat
Caesar salad dressing

MIDAFTERNOON SNACK

Whey protein shake

DINNER

4 ounces grilled or broiled lean hamburger patty

1 sliced tomato

1 cup cooked wild rice

POSTDINNER

1 cup decaf green tea mixed with a favorite herbal tea

(Day 17)

BREAKFAST

1 cup oatmeal with 2 tablespoons walnuts or sunflower seeds sprinkled on top,
sweetened with cinnamon and Truvia

1 pear

MIDMORNING SNACK

Whey protein shake

LUNCH

Tuna salad on lettuce and sliced tomato: 2 cans (3 ounces each for a total of 6 ounces) water-packed tuna mixed with ¼ cup chopped celery, 2 tablespoons chopped onion, and 1 tablespoon low-fat mayonnaise

1 cup fresh blueberries or other berries in season

MIDAFTERNOON SNACK

2 boiled eggs

DINNER

Dinner out at a Mexican restaurant: fajita steak strips (the size of your palm) with bell peppers, onions, and seasoning

1 cup brown rice topped with salsa

POSTDINNER

1 cup decaf green tea mixed with a favorite herbal tea

(Day 18)

BREAKFAST

Whey protein shake with 1 cup frozen spinach and 1 cup frozen berries

MIDMORNING SNACK

2 tablespoons raw almond butter with 3 celery sticks

LUNCH

1 cup beans (kidney beans, black beans, garbanzo beans, etc.) rolled in 2 whole wheat tortillas, topped with salsa

1 cup grilled bell peppers

MIDAFTERNOON SNACK

½ avocado with salt (optional)

DINNER

4 ounces grilled chicken

1 cup brown rice or wild rice

1 cup steamed greens (spinach, mustard greens, turnip greens, etc.)

POSTDINNER

1 cup decaf green tea mixed with a favorite herbal tea

Day 19

BREAKFAST

1 cup quinoa, sweetened with Truvia

1 cup mixed berries

MIDMORNING SNACK

1 cup Greek-style yogurt

LUNCH

4 ounces baked or grilled chicken

1 cup vegetarian vegetable soup

1 small apple

MIDAFTERNOON SNACK

Whey protein shake

DINNER

4 ounces grilled salmon

1 cup brown rice

1 cup chopped cucumber mixed with ½ cup cubed tomatoes tossed
with 1 tablespoon olive oil & 1 teaspoon balsamic vinegar

POSTDINNER

1 cup decaf green tea mixed with a favorite herbal tea

Day 20

BREAKFAST

1 cup oatmeal

1 sliced apple or peach

MIDMORNING SNACK

1 cup low-fat cottage cheese

LUNCH

Cheese melt: 1 ounce low-fat cheddar cheese melted on 1 slice
whole wheat bread with 1 sliced tomato

1 cup chopped fresh pineapple

MIDAFTERNOON SNACK

1 cup Greek-style yogurt

DINNER

4 ounces grilled flank steak

1 baked sweet potato with 1 pat butter

1 cup steamed spinach or other green vegetable

POSTDINNER

1 cup decaf green tea mixed with a favorite herbal tea

Day 21

BREAKFAST

1 slice whole wheat bread spread with ¼ cup part-skim ricotta cheese

1 cup mango slices

MIDMORNING SNACK

¾ cup low-fat cottage cheese

LUNCH

4 ounces sliced roast turkey

1 cup steamed asparagus

1 cup red seedless grapes

MIDAFTERNOON SNACK

2 tablespoons nut butter with 3 celery slices

DINNER

4 ounces baked cod

1 cup grilled eggplant

1 cup brown rice

POSTDINNER

1 cup decaf green tea mixed with a favorite herbal tea

(Day 22)

BREAKFAST

1 cup Greek-Style yogurt

1 cup tropical fruit compote: mixed pineapple, kiwi, and papaya cubes

MIDMORNING SNACK

Whey protein shake blended with 1 handful fresh spinach

LUNCH

1 cup bean soup

1 slice whole wheat bread

1 cup tossed salad with 2 tablespoons low-calorie salad dressing

MIDAFTERNOON SNACK

1 apple

DINNER

4 ounces grilled boneless pork loin or lamb chop

1 cup steamed broccoli

1 baked sweet potato

1 cup brown rice

POSTDINNER

1 cup decaf green tea mixed with a favorite herbal tea

(**Day 23**)

BREAKFAST

1 slice whole wheat toast

1 ounce low-fat cheddar cheese

2 slices tomato

MIDMORNING SNACK

1 cup Greek-style yogurt

1 cup sliced fresh strawberries

LUNCH

Roast beef wrap: 4 ounces lean roast beef rolled in 1 whole wheat tortilla
with ½ cup shredded carrots, 1 lettuce leaf, and 2 tablespoons ranch
or Thousand Island dressing

1 cup red and yellow bell pepper strips

MIDAFTERNOON SNACK

1 banana

DINNER

4 ounces grilled chicken

1 cup steamed zucchini and yellow squash

POSTDINNER

1 cup decaf green tea mixed with a favorite herbal tea

(**Day 24**)

BREAKFAST

1 cup oatmeal

2 boiled eggs

MIDMORNING SNACK

Whey protein shake blended with 1 frozen chopped banana

LUNCH

4 ounces baked halibut

1 large tossed salad with 2 tablespoons salad dressing

2 small plums

MIDAFTERNOON SNACK

1 cup chopped assorted veggies dipped in salsa

DINNER

1 baked Cornish game hen, skin removed

1 cup cooked wild rice

1 cup broccoli steamed with red bell pepper strips

POSTDINNER

1 cup decaf green tea mixed with a favorite herbal tea

(**Day 25**)

BREAKFAST

1 cup oat bran

1 cup fresh blueberries or blackberries

MIDMORNING SNACK

Whey protein shake blended with 1 handful frozen spinach

LUNCH

Quick pizza: 1 whole wheat pita topped with ½ cup marinara sauce, ¼ cup
part-skim mozzarella cheese, and 2 slices zucchini, broiled until cheese melts

1 cup tossed salad with 2 tablespoons low-calorie Italian dressing

1 cup green seedless grapes

MIDAFTERNOON SNACK

1 cup chopped assorted veggies dipped in salsa

DINNER

4 ounces grilled tuna steak

1 cup steamed broccoli

1 sliced fresh tomato topped with basil leaves and sprinkled with balsamic
vinegar

POSTDINNER

1 cup decaf green tea mixed with a favorite herbal tea

(Day 26)

BREAKFAST

Whey protein shake blended with 1 cup fresh or frozen blueberries

1 slice whole wheat bread with 1 pat butter

MIDMORNING SNACK

2 tablespoons nut butter with 3 celery slices

LUNCH

1 cup lentil soup

Tomato and zucchini salad (½ cup each chopped tomatoes and zucchini cubes,
drizzled with 1 tablespoon balsamic vinegar)

MIDAFTERNOON SNACK

1 cup fresh mango chunks

DINNER

4 ounces grilled scallops

1 cup cooked quinoa

½ acorn squash, baked and sprinkled with cinnamon and Truvia

POSTDINNER

1 cup decaf green tea mixed with a favorite herbal tea

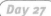 **Day 27**

BREAKFAST

1 cup low-fat cottage cheese

1 banana

MIDMORNING SNACK

1 apple

10 almonds

LUNCH

4 ounces roast pork tenderloin

1 cup brown rice

1 cup steamed asparagus

MIDAFTERNOON SNACK

Whey protein shake

DINNER

4 ounces turkey burger (made with lean ground turkey) served open face
on 1 slice whole wheat toast

1 cup cabbage salad (1 cup green or red cabbage with ¼ cup shredded carrots,
tossed with 1 tablespoon low-calorie slaw dressing)

POSTDINNER

1 cup decaf green tea mixed with a favorite herbal tea

(Day 28)

Breakfast

1 cup oatmeal cooked with 1 grated apple and flavored with cinnamon
and Truvia

Midmorning Snack

2 boiled eggs

Lunch

4 ounces grilled chicken breast

1 cup whole wheat couscous

1 cup tossed salad (lettuce, carrots, and grape tomatoes, tossed
with 2 tablespoons reduced-fat Thousand Island dressing)

Midafternoon Snack

1 nectarine

Dinner

4 ounces baked perch fillet

1 cup beans (kidney beans, black beans, garbanzo beans, etc.)

1 cup steamed broccoli or cauliflower

Postdinner

1 cup decaf green tea mixed with a favorite herbal tea

(Day 29)

Breakfast

2 boiled eggs

1 cup mixed berries

Midmorning Snack

1 cup Greek-style yogurt

LUNCH

4 ounces sliced roast beef on 2 slices whole wheat bread with brown mustard

1 sliced tomato

1 apple

MIDAFTERNOON SNACK

1 cup chopped veggies dipped in salsa

DINNER

4 ounces baked turkey breast

1 baked sweet potato

1 cup steamed mixed vegetables

POSTDINNER

1 cup decaf green tea mixed with a favorite herbal tea

(Day 30)

BREAKFAST

1 cup Greek-style yogurt

1 cup sliced strawberries

MIDMORNING SNACK

Whey protein shake blended with 1 handful fresh spinach

LUNCH

Tuna pocket sandwich: (3 ounces canned tuna mixed with 2 tablespoons reduced-fat mayonnaise, 2 tablespoons each minced onion, celery, and grated carrot), 1 lettuce leaf, 1 ounce reduced-fat swiss cheese in whole wheat pita bread

MIDAFTERNOON SNACK

1 apple, pear, or peach

DINNER

    4 ounces grilled salmon

    1 cup romaine lettuce tossed with tomatoes, fresh zucchini,
        and 2 tablespoons fat-free Caesar dressing

    1 cup brown rice

POSTDINNER

    1 cup decaf green tea mixed with a favorite herbal tea

(Day 31)

BREAKFAST

    2 boiled eggs

    1 cup oatmeal

    ½ grapefruit

MIDMORNING SNACK

    Yogurt parfait: 1 cup Greek-style yogurt, layered with sliced banana

LUNCH

    1 cup tomato soup, prepared with water

    1 ounce low-calorie cheese

    6 whole wheat crackers

MIDAFTERNOON SNACK

    ½ avocado, sliced, and 1 cup chopped assorted veggies

DINNER

    4 ounces grilled shrimp

    Garbanzo bean salad: 1 cup garbanzo beans on a generous bed of lettuce,
        drizzled with 1 tablespoon olive oil & 2 tablespoons balsamic vinegar

    1 cup steamed asparagus

POSTDINNER

    1 cup decaf green tea mixed with a favorite herbal tea

Hot and Healthy Recipes

This section is stocked with sixty gourmet-quality recipes, courtesy of Sunfare—a company I love whose healthy delicious meals make up a proper nutritional breakdown. You may mix and match the recipes at your discretion within the following guidelines:

* Eat five times per day in this order: breakfast, midmorning snack, lunch, midafternoon snack, dinner.

* Eat every three to four hours.

* Breakfast may only come from the breakfast recipes.

* Lunch and dinner recipes can be interchanged; lunch and dinner cannot come from the breakfast recipes.

* The portion sizes of the plan recipes are calculated for a daily intake of fifteen hundred calories.

* Each recipe serves one person, except for the rice recipes—serving sizes of these are indicated under "sides."

* The sugar totals indicated are per meal.

Tips for the Healthy Chef

A few simple changes in how you prepare your food will help to clean it up so that you're always eating the healthiest version of a meal:

* It's best to grill meat, so that its fat releases and drips away.

* When baking fish, use the same process: Bake until the natural juices or "fats" begin to release from the meat; this is also an excellent method to determine doneness.

* Never fry.

* Zucchini, squash, and eggplant can be sliced thin to layer lasagna.

* Substitute cauliflower for mashed potatoes by boiling and mashing to the desired consistency.

* Use low-fat cheese and reduced-fat salad dressings.

* When using ground turkey, use ground turkey breast.

* Replace vegetables sautéed in butter with steamed or roasted vegetables.

* Roast vegetables on a cookie sheet with a touch of Mrs. Dash for a flavorful preparation.

* Green, red, and yellow bell peppers cut up are similar to chips, and great with a low-fat dip or guacamole.

* If you're craving an evening snack, have a cup of fresh berries (blueberries, blackberries, raspberries, strawberries).

* Use olive oil instead of canola or vegetable oil.

* If you're sautéing, use olive oil instead of butter, and coated, nonstick pans. Monitor usage by putting olive oil in a clean spray bottle; just a couple of squirts is adequate, and will coat the bottom of a sauté pan evenly.

* Avoid white flour and refined sugar altogether; use Truvia as a sweetener.

* If you're adding a starch to a meal, make sure it is whole grain or whole wheat.

* Add flavor with fresh herbs.

Tips for Accelerated Weight Loss

* Excessive dairy can add a layer of fat to the body, which decreases muscle tone.

* Alcohol is a form of carbohydrate high in sugar; the less sugar you have in your system, the better your chance for fat loss. Alcohol also slows down the metabolism and dehydrates the body of essential fluids.

* Sauces generally start with oil and/or butter (fat)—and fat adds calories. The more calories you consume, the lower your chances of burning fat.

Breakfast

Chocolate Oatmeal

Calories: 418

INGREDIENTS:

2 cups water

1¼ cups instant oatmeal

½ cup low-sugar chocolate protein
   powder

Recipe courtesy: Sunfare

PREPARATION:

Bring the water to a boil on the
stove or in the microwave. Add the
oatmeal and protein powder into
the pot. Cool, and scoop into balls,
and serve.

SIDE:

1 cup mixed frozen berries

SUGARS: 5.6 grams

Cottage Cheese Parfait

Calories: 409

INGREDIENTS:

2 tsp. sunflower seeds

2 tsp. slivered almonds

2 tbsp. low-sugar granola

1½ cups low-fat cottage cheese

3 each large sliced strawberries

10 each raspberries

Recipe courtesy: Sunfare

PREPARATION:

Toss together the nuts and the
granola. Place the mixture in
the bottom of a container. Scoop
the cottage cheese into balls and
place on top of the mixture. Top
with the berries and serve.

SUGARS: 6.4 grams

American Omelet

Calories: 406

INGREDIENTS:

1 oz. turkey ham, diced

Salt and pepper to taste

2 eggs

2 oz. low-fat cheddar cheese

Recipe courtesy: Sunfare

PREPARATION:

Sauté the turkey ham and season with salt and pepper. Once the turkey ham has caramelized, add the egg and cook until set. Fold the egg to form an omelet and top with low-fat cheddar cheese.

SIDES:

½ cup blueberries (approx. 50 berries)

1 slice whole-grain toast

SUGARS: 5.9 grams

Breakfast Hash

Calories: 393

INGREDIENTS:

1 oz. turkey ham

Salt and pepper to taste

2 eggs

1 oz. part-skim mozzarella cheese, shredded

Recipe courtesy: Sunfare

PREPARATION:

Sauté the turkey ham and season with salt and pepper. Once the turkey ham is caramelized, add the eggs and scramble. Place on a plate and top with the cheese.

SIDES:

½ wedge honeydew

1 slice whole-grain toast

SUGARS: 8.1 grams

Burrito Italiano

Calories: 378

INGREDIENTS:

2 eggs

½ cup chopped fresh spinach leaves

½ red bell pepper, roasted

1 oz. mozzarella cheese, part skim (shredded)

Salt and pepper to taste

1 10-inch whole wheat low-carb tortilla

PREPARATION:

Scramble the eggs in a pan. When they're almost done, add the spinach, bell pepper, and cheese. Season with salt and pepper. When the cheese has melted, wrap in a burrito.

SUGARS: 1.7 grams

Recipe courtesy: Sunfare

Egg Sandwich with Canadian Bacon

Calories: 406

INGREDIENTS:

2 medium-size eggs

1 tsp. olive oil

1 oz. Canadian bacon

2 cups fresh spinach leaves

1 oz. Parmesan cheese

Recipe courtesy: Sunfare

PREPARATION:

Fry the eggs in a sauté pan with the oil until they reach your desired doneness. Grill the Canadian bacon. Lay the spinach as a base and top with Canadian bacon first, then the fried eggs. Top with Parmesan cheese.

SIDE:

½ slice whole wheat English muffin

SUGARS: 0.6 gram

Goat Cheese and Tomato Basil Omelet

Calories: 387

INGREDIENTS:

¼ cup chopped tomatoes

2 tbsp. chopped basil

2 medium-size eggs

½ oz. goat cheese, crumbled

Recipe courtesy: Sunfare

PREPARATION:

Mix the chopped tomatoes and basil with the eggs. Cook the omelet and top with goat cheese crumbles.

SIDES:

½ grapefruit

Truvia or stevia sweetener

1 slice 100% whole-grain sugar-free toast

SUGARS: 8.25 grams

Scrambled Eggs with Cheese

Calories: 421

INGREDIENTS:

2 eggs

1 tsp. olive oil

½ cup diced tomato

1 oz. low-fat cheddar cheese

Recipe courtesy: Sunfare

PREPARATION:

Scramble the eggs in a skillet with the oil and tomato until done. Top with the cheddar cheese.

SIDES:

1 cup kiwi fruit

1 slice 100% whole-grain sugar-free toast

SUGARS: 8.4 grams

Italian Omelet

Calories: 415

INGREDIENTS:

1½ oz. Italian chicken sausage

2 tbsp. diced onions

2 tbsp. diced bell peppers

2 tbsp. diced tomatoes

Salt and pepper to taste

2 medium eggs

1 tbsp. chiffonade basil

½ oz. part-skim mozzarella cheese, shredded

Chives, for garnish

Recipe courtesy: Sunfare

PREPARATION:

Dice the Italian chicken sausage. Sauté the onions and peppers, then add the sausage. Toss in the tomatoes and adjust the seasoning with salt and pepper.

Add the eggs and basil. Cook, then fold into an omelet. Sprinkle with the mozzarella and serve with chives as a garnish.

SIDES:

3 each large strawberries

½ slice whole wheat English muffin

SUGARS: 4.9 grams

Skillet Scramble

Calories: 399

INGREDIENTS:

2 oz. chicken, diced

3–4 broccoli florets, trimmed

2 medium eggs

Salt and pepper to taste

1 oz. low-fat cheddar cheese, shredded

Recipe courtesy: Sunfare

PREPARATION:

Sauté the chicken. When it's almost done, add the broccoli. Add the eggs and continue cooking until done. Season with salt and pepper and top with cheddar cheese.

SIDES:

1 cup grapes

1 slice 100% whole grain sugar-free toast

SUGARS:

8.6 grams

Mozzarella, Spinach, and Pepper Omelet

Calories: 391

INGREDIENTS:

 2 medium eggs

 ¼ cup diced bell peppers

 ¼ cup diced onions

 ½ whole wheat English muffin

 1 oz. part-skim mozzarella cheese,
   shredded

 ½ cup fresh spinach leaves

Recipe courtesy: Sunfare

PREPARATION:

Preheat the oven to 350°F.
Combine whole eggs.

Sauté the bell peppers and onions.

Pour the egg mixture over the
peppers and onions. Cook the
omelet.

Place the ½ English muffin on a
baking sheet, sprinkle with the
cheese, and melt in the oven.

Top with the spinach and a
portioned amount of the omelet.
This will be open-faced!

SIDE:

3 large strawberries

SUGARS: 4.7 grams

Breakfast Caprese with Pesto Sauce

Calories: 406

INGREDIENTS:

 ¼ cup sliced mushrooms

 ¼ cup chopped red onions

 3 eggs

 2 tbsp. pesto, on the side

 2 slices tomato

Recipe courtesy: Sunfare

PREPARATION:

Sauté the mushrooms and onions.
Pour in the eggs and cook until
firm. Plate with tomato and pesto.

SIDES:

3 large strawberries

Truvia or stevia sweetener

1 slice 100% whole-grain sugar-free toast

SUGARS: 5.7 grams

Scrambled Eggs with Goat Cheese and Dill

Calories: 376

INGREDIENTS:

2 eggs

Salt and pepper to taste

2 tbsp. chopped dill

1 oz. goat cheese, crumbled

Recipe courtesy: Sunfare

PREPARATION:

Scramble the eggs and season with salt and pepper. Add the dill and cook for 1 additional minute. Top with crumbled goat cheese.

SIDES:

1 cup grapes

1 slice 100% whole-grain sugar-free toast

SUGARS: 4.85 grams

Mushroom, Pepper, and Fontina Omelet

Calories: 405

INGREDIENTS:

2 tbsp. diced red bell peppers

2 tbsp. diced green bell peppers

¼ cup diced shiitake mushrooms

2 large eggs

1 oz. Fontina cheese

Pinch of parsley, for garnish

Recipe courtesy: Sunfare

PREPARATION:

Sauté the red and green bell peppers with the mushrooms. Add the eggs and cook. Fold the omelet and serve with a slice of Fontina cheese. Garnish with a sprig of parsley.

SIDES:

1 cup watermelon

1 slice 100% whole-grain sugar-free toast

SUGARS: 8.62 grams

Open-Faced Breakfast Quesadilla with Chicken

Calories: 394

INGREDIENTS:

3 oz. chicken breast (in strips)

Taco seasoning, to taste

½ oz. low-fat cheddar cheese, shredded

½ oz. part-skim mozzarella cheese, shredded

1 6-inch whole wheat tortilla

Chopped cilantro to taste

¼ cup salsa, on the side

PREPARATION:

Season the chicken breast with taco seasoning. Grill it and cut into strips. Blend the two cheeses.

On a small tortilla, place some cheese; top with strips of chicken, more cheese, and cilantro. Serve with salsa.

SUGARS: 2.61 grams

Recipe courtesy: Sunfare

Sausage and Egg Scramble

Calories: 421

INGREDIENTS:

2 oz. chicken sausage

Salt and pepper to taste

2 medium eggs

1 oz. part-skim mozzarella cheese, shredded

¼ cup Mexican salsa

Recipe courtesy: Sunfare

PREPARATION:

Sauté the chicken sausage and season with salt and pepper.

Add the eggs and scramble.

Place on a plate and top with cheese.

Serve with salsa on the side.

SIDES:

1 cup pineapple

1 slice 100% whole-grain sugar-free toast

SUGARS: 7.81 grams

Sausage Mushroom Scramble

Calories: 397

INGREDIENTS:

2 oz. Italian chicken sausage, diced

½ cup shiitake mushrooms

¼ cup chopped tomatoes

Whites of 4 eggs

1 oz. Parmesan cheese

Recipe courtesy: Sunfare

PREPARATION:

Sauté the sausage. Add the mushrooms and tomatoes, sautéing the mixture together. Add the egg whites and scramble. Top with Parmesan cheese.

SIDES:

1 cup grapes

1 slice 100% whole-grain sugar-free toast

SUGARS: 5.51 grams

Spinach and Feta Omelet

Calories: 387

INGREDIENTS:

½ cup fresh spinach leaves

3 eggs

2 oz. feta, crumbled

Recipe courtesy: Sunfare

PREPARATION:

Sauté the spinach. Add the eggs and cook. Fold the cooked omelet and garnish with feta crumbles.

SIDES:

½ cup watermelon

½ slice whole wheat English muffin

SUGARS: 7.3 grams

Green Energy Protein Shake

INGREDIENTS:

1 scoop whey isolate powder

2 cups frozen spinach

1 banana

1 tbsp. lemon juice

Ice water

Recommended daily allowance
  glutamine powder

Recommended daily allowance BCAAs
  powder

Recommended daily allowance flaxseed oil

PREPARATION:

Mix all ingredients in a blender.
Serve.

Recipe Courtesy: Sunfare

Citrus Power Cleanse Protein Shake

INGREDIENTS:

1 grapefruit

1 tbsp. ginger

1 scoop whey powder

Ice water

Recommended daily allowance
  glutamine powder

Recommended daily allowance BCAAs
  powder

Recommended daily allowance flaxseed oil

PREPARATION:

Mix all ingredients in a blender.
Serve.

Recipe Courtesy: Sunfare

Slim Berry Delight Protein Shake

INGREDIENTS:

1 cup frozen mixed berries

1 scoop whey powder

1 cup frozen spinach

Ice water (up to 12oz)

Recommended daily allowance
    glutamine powder

Recommended daily allowance BCAAs
    powder

Recommended daily allowance flaxseed oil

PREPARATION:

Mix all ingredients in a blender.
Serve.

Recipe Courtesy: Sunfare

Lunch

Asian-Style Stir-Fry

Calories: 420

INGREDIENTS:

3 oz. filet mignon

Salt and pepper to taste

¼ red bell pepper, diced

4 broccoli florets

1 oz. diced onions

6 individual snow peas

3 each shiitake mushrooms

1 tsp. soy sauce

1 tbsp. orange juice

½ tsp. minced ginger

⅛ tsp. sesame seeds

PREPARATION:

Clean and cut the filet into slices.
Season with salt and pepper, then
sauté. Remove from the pan and
reserve. In the same sauté pan, stir-
fry all the vegetables.

Whisk together the soy sauce,
orange juice, and ginger. Add this
mixture to the sauté pan along with
the reserved beef. Add seeds. Serve.

SIDE:

¼ cup brown rice

SUGARS: 6.1 grams

Recipe courtesy: Sunfare

Cajun Fish Tacos

Calories: 379

INGREDIENTS:

4 oz. bass fillet

Cajun seasoning

2 large leaves butter leaf lettuce

2 oz. shredded cabbage

1 oz. low-fat cheddar cheese, shredded

2 oz. julienned tomatoes

2 oz. black beans

¼ cup salsa

Recipe courtesy: Sunfare

PREPARATION:

Coat the fish with Cajun seasoning and place on a sheet pan. Bake in a 300°F oven for 12 to 18 minutes or until done. Drain the excess juice and transfer the fish to a clean sheet before cooling.

Cut fillet into 2 pieces. Wrap the fish in the lettuce leaves with the cabbage, cheese, and tomatoes.

Serve with a side of black beans and salsa.

SIDES:

4 oz. steamed broccoli

¼ cup Mexican rice

SUGARS: 6.2 grams

Garlic-Crusted Roughy

Calories: 378

INGREDIENTS:

6 oz. roughy fillet

2 tbsp. finely chopped garlic

1 tsp. or spray olive oil

Parsley to taste

Paprika to taste

For the Sauce:

⅔ cup chopped red bell peppers

¼ cup chicken stock

Salt and pepper to taste

Recipe courtesy: Sunfare

PREPARATION:

Preheat the oven to 350°F.

Marinate the roughy with the garlic, olive oil, parsley, and paprika. Sear the fish on one side, then bake in the oven 10–15 minutes or until done.

For the Sauce:

Puree the red peppers and chicken stock. Season with salt and pepper to taste and serve on the side.

SIDES:

1 cup brussels sprouts

¼ cup brown rice pilaf

SUGARS: 6.7 grams

Asian Turkey Lettuce Wraps

Calories: 395

INGREDIENTS:

1 oz. diced roasted red bell pepper

1 oz. sliced cucumbers

½ oz. diced raw onions

½ oz. bean sprouts

3 cherry tomatoes, cut in half

¼ cup shredded carrots

4 oz. turkey tenders, diced

1 oz. peanut sauce

3 lettuce leaves

For the Sauce:

¼ cup low-calorie peanut butter

2 tsp. low-sodium soy sauce

1 tbsp. brown sugar Splenda

1 tbsp. fresh lemon juice

1 clove garlic, minced

¼ cup coconut milk

¼ cup water

Red chili flakes to taste

Recipe courtesy: Sunfare

PREPARATION:

Mix all of the vegetables. Sauté the turkey tenders with the peanut sauce. Serve in lettuce leaves with mixed vegetables.

For the Sauce:

Add all ingredients in a blender and blend to a smooth texture. (Yields 4 servings.)

SIDE:

2 oz. fried brown rice

SUGARS: 8.85 grams

Grilled Scampi Bowl

Calories: 403

INGREDIENTS:

¼ red onion, sliced

6–7 whole asparagus

5 large shrimp, tail on

3–4 pieces hearts of palm

⅓ cup diced tomatoes

Lemon wedge, for garnish

Recipe courtesy: Sunfare

PREPARATION:

Grill the red onions and asparagus, then the shrimp. Toss the shrimp with grilled onions, asparagus, hearts of palm, and diced tomato. Garnish with a lemon wedge.

SIDE:

¼ cup wild rice

SUGARS: 6.5 grams

Chicken Quesadilla

Calories: 398

INGREDIENTS:

3 oz. chicken breast

Taco seasoning to taste

¼ oz. part-skim mozzarella cheese, grated

¼ oz. low-fat cheddar cheese, grated

1 oz. black beans

1 6-inch whole wheat low-carb tortilla

¼ cup Mexican salsa

Chopped cilantro to taste

Recipe courtesy: Sunfare

PREPARATION:

Season the chicken with the taco seasoning and grill. Chop the grilled chicken, put it in a sauté pan, and add the cheeses and beans. Cook until heated through. Sprinkle cilantro on top.

Put the mixture on a whole wheat tortilla and serve with Mexican salsa on the side.

SIDE:

4 oz. grilled asparagus

SUGARS: 4.28 grams

Grilled Vegetable Chicken Bowl

Calories: 382

INGREDIENTS:

4 oz. chicken breast

Lemon pepper to taste

Onion powder to taste

3–4 asparagus spears, sliced

1½ oz. summer squash, chopped

1 oz. julienned red bell pepper

1 oz. diced eggplant

1½ oz. diced zucchini

3 each chopped sun-dried tomatoes

6–7 whole cherry tomatoes

2 oz. balsamic vinaigrette

PREPARATION:

Season the chicken breast with lemon pepper and onion powder. Grill it on both sides, then cut it into slices.

Season the vegetables with lemon pepper and onion powder, then grill.

Reduce the balsamic vinaigrette in a sauté pan and serve on the side.

SIDE:

½ cup brown rice

SUGARS: 6.84 grams

Recipe courtesy: Sunfare

Thai Pork and Basil Stir-Fry

(*Calories: 426*)

INGREDIENTS:

   4 oz. pork tenderloin

   2 tsp. soy sauce

   1 tbsp. sherry vinegar

   2 tsp. roasted sesame oil

   2 tbsp. garlic

   4 leaves whole basil (2 tbsp. chiffonade)

   2 tbsp. minced cilantro

   1 tbsp. red pepper flakes

   6 snow peas, cut in half and trimmed

   4 whole grape tomatoes

   2 each julienned shiitake mushrooms

   1 oz. shredded carrots

PREPARATION:

Cut the pork into thin medallions. Whisk together the soy sauce, vinegar, oil, garlic, basil, cilantro, and red pepper flakes. Then let the pork sit in this marinade for an hour.

Sauté the pork with the marinade until done. Set aside.

Sauté the vegetables until nearly done, then toss them with the pork.

SIDE:

½ cup fried brown rice

SUGARS: 8.62 grams

Recipe courtesy: Sunfare

Italian Stuffed Chicken

Calories: 409

INGREDIENTS:

¼ cup sliced mushrooms

⅓ cup fresh spinach leaves

2 each chopped kalamata olives

½ oz. grated Parmesan cheese

1 tsp. olive oil

4 oz. chicken breast

Pinch of paprika

2 oz. marinara sauce

Recipe courtesy: Sunfare

PREPARATION:

Preheat the oven to 350°F. Sauté the mushrooms and spinach. Add the olives, Parmesan cheese, and olive oil.

Pound the chicken flat, top with the olive-mushroom mixture, then roll it up while tucking in the sides. Sprinkle with paprika, then bake 15–18 minutes or until done. Serve on top of marinara sauce.

SIDES:

4 oz. yellow wax beans

2 oz. whole wheat bowtie pasta

SUGARS: 7 grams

Jalapeño Cheese Turkey Burgers

Calories: 406

INGREDIENTS:

5 oz. ground turkey

1 tsp. chopped parsley

Garlic to taste

Salt and pepper to taste

¼ jalapeño pepper, seeded and chopped

1 oz. Jack cheese, shredded

Recipe courtesy: Sunfare

PREPARATION:

In a bowl, combine the first three ingredients. Salt and pepper to taste.

Mix the jalapeños and the Jack cheese; set aside.

Portion out 2 patties; make an indentation in the middle of each patty and stuff with the cheese mixture. Grill the burgers.

SIDES:

¼ cup pineapple

½ whole wheat hamburger bun

SUGARS: 5.1 grams

Oriental Chicken Stir-Fry

Calories: 353

INGREDIENTS:

3–4 broccoli florets

¼ cup diced onions

¼ red bell pepper, julienned

5 oz. chicken breast, diced

1 tsp. soy sauce

1 tsp. or spray olive oil

⅓ cup bean sprouts

Recipe courtesy: Sunfare

PREPARATION:

Blanch the broccoli until al dente; set aside.

Sauté the onions until slightly caramelized; set aside.

Sauté the bell peppers and set aside.

Marinate the chicken in the soy sauce. In a very hot skillet, heat olive oil and sauté the chicken until done. Add the vegetables and serve.

SIDE:

½ cup brown rice

SUGARS: 8.83 grams

Soft Taco

Calories: 381

INGREDIENTS:

4 oz. chicken breast, cut into strips

Cayenne pepper to taste

Salt and pepper to taste

6 leaves butter leaf lettuce

1 oz. shredded cabbage

1 oz. sliced radishes

1 tsp. black beans

1 oz. low-fat cheddar cheese, shredded

2 oz. salsa

Recipe courtesy: Sunfare

PREPARATION:

Sauté the chicken with cayenne pepper, salt, and pepper until done. Place the chicken in the butter leaf lettuce and top with the rest of the ingredients, cheese on top. Serve with a side of salsa.

SIDES:

¼ cup pineapple

2 oz. Mexican rice

SUGARS: 8.53 grams

Teriyaki Tuna

Calories: 424

INGREDIENTS:

6 each sliced snow peas

2 oz. julienned radishes

2 oz. carrots, sliced

6 oz. ahi tuna, sliced

1 tsp. or spray olive oil

Salt and pepper to taste

1 tsp. black sesame seeds

2 tbsp. chopped green onions

1 oz. ponzu sauce

1 tsp. wasabi

Recipe courtesy: Sunfare

PREPARATION:

Blanch the snow peas, radishes, and carrots; set aside.

Coat the tuna with olive oil, salt and pepper, and sesame seeds. Then sear on all sides.

Place the green onions in the ponzu sauce. Cut the tuna and serve on top of the vegetables with a side of ponzu and wasabi.

SIDES:

1 cup roasted eggplant, asparagus, and yellow pepper

¼ cup brown rice

SUGARS: 8.31 grams

Turkey Meatballs

Calories: 424

INGREDIENTS:

4 oz. ground turkey

1 oz. finely chopped onions

2 tbsp. finely chopped parsley

1 oz. Parmesan cheese, shredded

1 medium egg

1 tsp. minced garlic

¼ cup marinara sauce

Recipe courtesy: Sunfare

PREPARATION:

Preheat the oven to 350°F.

Mix together the turkey, onions, parsley, cheese, egg, and garlic. Form into balls and place on a baking sheet. Bake 10–15 minutes or until done. Serve with marinara sauce.

SIDES:

2 cups asparagus

¼ cup whole wheat penne pasta

SUGARS: 8.33 grams

Thai Beef Stir-Fry

Calories: 414

INGREDIENTS:

3 oz. beef fillet

1 oz. low-sodium stir-fry sauce

3–4 broccoli florets

1 oz. sliced onions

⅓ yellow bell pepper, julienned

1 oz. bean sprouts

2 oz. snow peas

3 each sliced shiitake mushrooms

3 whole cherry tomatoes

¼ cup chopped cilantro

Recipe courtesy: Sunfare

PREPARATION:

Cut the beef into 2-inch strips and marinate in the stir-fry sauce. For best results, marinate for 1 hour.

Blanch all vegetables in boiling water and set aside.

Add the marinated beef to a hot sauté pan and sauté it quickly so as not to overcook. Add in vegetables and cook for 2 minutes. Place on a platter and top with fresh cilantro.

SIDE:

¼ cup brown rice

SUGARS: 8.65 grams

Dinner

Baja Beef Tacos

Calories: 418

INGREDIENTS:

3 oz. beef fillet

Salt and pepper to taste

¼ cup diced yellow peppers

¼ cup diced onions

1 tbsp. diced scallions

1 tsp. or spray olive oil

2 tbsp. pineapple juice

2 tbsp. chicken stock

6 romaine hearts

2 tbsp. salsa

1 oz. Mexican blend cheese (low-fat cheddar and part-skim mozzarella)

½ cup black beans

⅓ cup diced tomatoes

Recipe courtesy: Sunfare

PREPARATION:

Season the beef with salt and pepper and sear in a large pan. Cool the meat and dice it into small pieces.

Sauté the bell pepper, onions, and scallions in olive oil until caramelized. Add the beef and cook for 1 to 2 minutes or until the meat reaches your desired doneness. Add the pineapple juice and chicken stock to the pan and allow it to reduce.

Serve the tacos with the romaine hearts, salsa, cheese, black beans, and tomatoes.

SIDE:

¼ cup Mexican rice

SUGARS:

8.35 grams

Beef & Broccoli Stir-Fry

Calories: 418

INGREDIENTS:

For the Marinade:

1 oz. soy sauce

1 tsp. roasted sesame oil

Black pepper to taste

For the Stir-Fry:

3 oz. filet mignon, sliced

1 oz. stir-fry sauce

3–4 broccoli florets

1 tsp. or spray olive oil

Recipe courtesy: Sunfare

PREPARATION:

Make the marinade by mixing the ingredients together. For best results, marinate the beef slices for 1 hour.

Cook the beef in the stir-fry sauce until it's done. In a separate pan, sauté the broccoli in olive oil to your desired doneness. Mix all ingredients together and serve.

SIDE:

¼ cup brown rice

SUGARS: 8.35 grams

Black Cod Belle Jerez

Calories: 368

INGREDIENTS:

¼ cup sherry

1 tsp. lemon pepper

½ cup sliced shiitake mushrooms

½ cup chopped tomatoes

2 tbsp. diced green onions

1 tsp. sesame seeds

6 oz. cod

Recipe courtesy: Sunfare

PREPARATION:

Mix the sherry and lemon pepper over medium-high heat. Reduce. Add the shiitake mushrooms and sauté. Finish by adding the tomatoes and green onions and a sprinkle of sesame seeds.

Pan-sear the cod and top with the sauce.

SIDE:

2 cups artichoke, green bean, and asparagus sauté

SUGARS: 6.84 grams

Black Pepper New York Steak

Calories: 370

INGREDIENTS:

4 oz. New York strip, trimmed

Salt and pepper to taste

1 tsp. paprika

½ cup sliced portobello mushrooms

1 tsp. minced rosemary

¼ cup Marsala

2 cloves garlic, roasted

Rosemary sprig, for garnish

Recipe courtesy: Sunfare

PREPARATION:

Season the beef with salt, pepper, and paprika. In a sauté pan, sear the beef until it's done. Remove the meat and set aside. In the same pan, sauté the mushrooms; add the rosemary. Deglaze with Marsala.

Add the garlic and allow the liquid to reduce.

Serve the sauce over the beef and garnish with a rosemary sprig.

SIDES:

2 cups steamed broccoli

½ cup roasted new potatoes

SUGARS: 8.8 grams

Cherry Tomato Salmon

Calories: 420

INGREDIENTS:

6 oz. salmon

2 tbsp. lemon juice

1 tbsp. mixed fresh herbs

2 tbsp. minced garlic

¼ cup herb vinaigrette

4 cherry tomatoes, cut in half

1 sprig fresh thyme, for garnish

Recipe courtesy: Sunfare

PREPARATION:

Season the salmon fillet with the lemon juice, fresh herb mixture, and garlic. Coat it with vinaigrette. Put the cherry tomatoes on the baking tray with the salmon, and bake at 325°F until done. Garnish with fresh thyme.

SIDES:

2 cups steamed broccoli

½ cup brown rice

SUGARS: 7.7 grams

Chicken Bruschetta

Calories: 395

INGREDIENTS:

4 oz. chicken, butterflied

1 tsp. olive oil

1 tsp. onion powder

1 tsp. chili powder

2 oz. diced Roma tomatoes

1 tbsp. chiffonade basil

2 tbsp. minced garlic

Salt and pepper to taste

Recipe courtesy: Sunfare

PREPARATION:

Season the chicken with olive oil, onion powder, and chili powder. Grill until done. Combine the tomatoes, basil, and minced garlic. Season with salt and pepper to taste and serve with the grilled chicken.

SIDES:

2 cups steamed asparagus

¼ cup brown rice

SUGARS: 5.33 grams

Dijon Baked Sea Bass

Calories: 411

INGREDIENTS:

6 oz. sea bass

Salt and pepper to taste

¼ cup Dijon mustard

¼ cup lemon juice

Parsley

2 oz. sliced zucchini

1 oz. onions

2 oz. diced tomato

1 tsp. chopped garlic

1 tsp. or spray olive oil

Recipe courtesy: Sunfare

PREPARATION:

Preheat the oven to 350°F. Season the sea bass with salt and pepper, rub with Dijon mustard and lemon juice, sprinkle with parsley, and bake 10–15 minutes or until done.

Meanwhile, toss the vegetables in olive oil and season with salt and pepper. Roast vegetables in the oven to desired doneness. Serve with the baked fish.

SIDES:

2 cups steamed broccoli and cauliflower

¼ cup Spanish rice

SUGARS: 8.4 grams

Grilled Filet Mignon

Calories: 420

INGREDIENTS:

4 oz. filet mignon

Montreal steak seasoning to taste

Recipe courtesy: Sunfare

PREPARATION:

Rub the filet with seasoning; grill to your desired doneness.

SIDES:

2 cups steamed broccoli

3 roasted small purple potatoes

SUGARS: 7.4 grams

Chicken Kebabs

Calories: 410

INGREDIENTS:

4 oz. chicken breast (cubed)

¼ cup lemon juice

1 oz. red onions, thinly sliced

1 tsp. paprika

1 tsp. Mrs. Dash

½ bell pepper, cut into 1-inch pieces

Recipe courtesy: Sunfare

PREPARATION:

Marinate the chicken in the lemon juice, red onions, and paprika. Season with Mrs. Dash and skewer with the bell peppers. Grill everything until done.

SIDES:

2 cups kale

½ cup purple potatoes

SUGARS: 3.8 grams

Halibut with Black Bean Relish

Calories: 416

INGREDIENTS:

5 oz. halibut

1 tsp. chopped fresh rosemary

1 tsp. chopped fresh dill

1 tsp. chopped fresh parsley

1 tsp. chopped fresh mint

For the Black Bean Relish:

1 tbsp. black beans

1 oz. red onions, minced

1 oz. tomato, diced

2 tbsp. lemon juice

1 tsp. cilantro

1 tsp. cumin

Salt and pepper to taste

PREPARATION:

Season the halibut with herbs. Grill to your desired doneness.

For the Black Bean Relish:

Combine all ingredients and spread over the fish once it's cooked.

SIDES:

2 cups roasted broccoli and mushrooms

¼ cup Mexican rice

SUGARS:

7.15 grams

Recipe courtesy: Sunfare

Spicy Herb Chicken

Calories: 382

INGREDIENTS:

4 oz. chicken breast, butterflied

1 tsp. paprika

1 tsp. onion powder

1 tsp. garlic powder

1 tsp. chili powder

Olive oil spray

For the Sauce:

¾ roasted red pepper

2 tbsp. chicken stock

1 tsp. lemon pepper

Recipe courtesy: Sunfare

PREPARATION:

Rub the chicken with dry seasonings and spray with olive oil. Grill until done.

For the Sauce:

Puree the roasted red pepper and stock; season with lemon pepper.

Heat and serve with the grilled chicken.

SIDES:

2 cups yellow and green beans sauté

½ cup wild rice

SUGARS: 4.7 grams

Herb-Crusted Salmon

Calories: 394

INGREDIENTS:

6 oz. salmon fillet

1 tsp. or spray olive oil

Lemon pepper

1 tbsp. chopped fresh basil

1 tbsp. chopped fresh dill

1 tbsp. chopped fresh parsley

Lemon wedge, for garnish

Recipe courtesy: Sunfare

PREPARATION:

Season the salmon fillet with olive oil, lemon pepper, and the fresh herb mixture. Grill until done. Garnish with a lemon wedge and serve.

SIDES:

2 cups kale sauté

½ cup brown rice

SUGARS: 1.4 grams

Shrimp and Chicken

Calories: 390

INGREDIENTS:

1 oz. diced tomatoes

2 tbsp. sliced green onions

2 tbsp. tequila

1 oz. orange juice

3 oz. chicken breast (strips)

2 whole shrimp

1 tsp. taco seasoning

1 tsp. chili powder

Recipe courtesy: Sunfare

PREPARATION:

Sauté the tomatoes and onions with the tequila and orange juice.

Prepare the chicken and shrimp separately: Season each with taco seasoning and chili powder, then sauté until golden brown.

Add the sauce and simmer for 2 to 3 minutes.

SIDES:

2 cups brussels sprouts and carrots roasted

¼ cup brown rice

SUGARS: 6.8 grams

Steak Fajitas

Calories: 388

INGREDIENTS:

4 oz. skirt steak fillet, cut into strips

¼ tsp. salt

¼ tsp. pepper

¼ tsp. cumin

⅛ julienned red bell pepper

⅛ julienned yellow bell pepper

1 oz. julienned white onions

1 tsp. garlic powder

¼ cup salsa

Recipe courtesy: Sunfare

PREPARATION:

Sauté the beef and season with salt, pepper, and cumin. Set aside.

Sauté the vegetables, sprinkle with garlic powder, and serve with the beef and a side of salsa.

SIDES:

2 cups grilled asparagus

¼ cup Mexican rice

SUGARS: 6.97 grams

Side Dishes

Steamed Broccoli

INGREDIENTS:

2 cups broccoli (trimmed to florets)

Salt and pepper to taste

Recipe courtesy: Sunfare

PREPARATION:

Boil water and season with salt and pepper. Add the broccoli and cook till tender. Serve.

SUGARS:

4.4 grams

Sautéed Brussels Sprouts

INGREDIENTS:

1 tsp. oil

2 cups brussels sprouts, cut into quarters

Salt and pepper to taste

Recipe courtesy: Sunfare

PREPARATION:

Put the oil in a sauté pan and heat briefly over a medium flame. Add the brussels sprouts, cook till tender, season with salt and pepper, and serve.

SUGARS: 5.6 grams

Grilled Asparagus

INGREDIENTS:

2 cups trimmed asparagus

1 tsp. or spray olive oil

1 tbsp. Montreal steak seasoning

Recipe courtesy: Sunfare

PREPARATION:

Coat the asparagus with olive oil and Montreal steak seasoning. Grill till tender and serve.

SUGARS: 4.8 grams

Steamed Yellow Wax Beans

INGREDIENTS:

2 cups yellow wax beans

Salt and pepper to taste

Recipe courtesy: Sunfare

PREPARATION:

Trim off the ends of the wax beans.

Boil water in a pot. Season with salt and pepper, add the wax beans, cook till tender, and serve.

SUGARS: 6 grams

Roasted Eggplant, Carrots, and Yellow Pepper

INGREDIENTS:

½ cup baby carrots

½ cup julienned yellow bell pepper

1 cup eggplant cut into half medallions

1 tbsp. chopped fresh garlic

1 tsp. olive oil

Salt and pepper to taste

Recipe courtesy: Sunfare

PREPARATION:

Preheat the oven to 350°F.

Toss the vegetables in fresh garlic, olive oil, salt, and pepper. Place in a baking pan and cover with foil. Bake 8–12 minutes, until the vegetables are tender, then remove the foil and bake for another 5 minutes.

SUGARS: 7.3 grams

Steamed Asparagus

INGREDIENTS:

Salt and pepper to taste

2 cups trimmed asparagus

Recipe courtesy: Sunfare

PREPARATION:

Boil water, season with salt and pepper, add the asparagus, and cook till tender.

SUGARS: 4.8 grams

Artichoke, Green Beans, and Asparagus Sauté

INGREDIENTS:

1 tsp. oil

½ cup green beans

1 cup trimmed asparagus

½ cup artichoke hearts

Salt and pepper to taste

Recipe courtesy: Sunfare

PREPARATION:

Put the oil in a sauté pan and heat briefly over a medium flame. Add the green beans, then the asparagus, then the artichoke hearts, till tender. Season with salt and pepper.

SUGARS: 5.2 grams

Steamed Broccoli and Cauliflower

INGREDIENTS:

Salt and pepper to taste

1 cup broccoli trimmed into florets

1 cup cauliflower trimmed into florets

Recipe courtesy: Sunfare

PREPARATION:

Boil water and season with salt and pepper. Add the broccoli and cauliflower and cook till tender.

SUGARS: 4.4 grams

Kale Sauté

INGREDIENTS:

3 cups chopped kale

1 tsp. olive oil

1 tsp. Montreal steak seasoning

Recipe courtesy: Sunfare

PREPARATION:

Put the kale in a pot and add water to cover. Simmer over a medium flame till dry. Repeat three more times. After the third final cooking, add the olive oil and Montreal steak seasoning. Continue cooking till tender.

SUGARS: 3.2 grams

Broccoli and Mushroom Sauté

INGREDIENTS:

1 tsp. olive oil

1 cup broccoli trimmed into florets

1 cup button mushrooms

Salt and pepper to taste

Recipe courtesy: Sunfare

PREPARATION:

Put the oil in a sauté pan and heat briefly over a medium flame. Add the broccoli and cook for 3 minutes. Add the mushrooms and continue cooking till the vegetables are tender. Season with salt and pepper.

SUGARS: 5.6 grams

Yellow and Green Bean Sauté

INGREDIENTS:

1 tsp. olive oil

1 cup trimmed green beans

1 cup trimmed yellow beans

1 tsp. Mrs. Dash

Recipe courtesy: Sunfare

PREPARATION:

Put the olive oil in a sauté pan and heat briefly over a medium flame. Add the beans and cook till tender. Add the Mrs. Dash and toss.

SUGARS: 3.2 grams

Roasted Carrots and Brussels Sprouts

INGREDIENTS:

1 cup brussels sprouts, cut in half

1 cup baby carrots

1 tsp. olive oil

1 tsp. Mrs. Dash

Recipe courtesy: Sunfare

PREPARATION:

Preheat the oven to 350°F. Toss the brussels sprouts and carrots in olive oil and Mrs. Dash. Place them in a baking pan and cover with foil; bake till tender. Remove the foil and continue baking for 5 more minutes, then serve.

SUGARS: 6.7 grams

Mexican Rice

INGREDIENTS:

1 tsp. oil

2 tbsp. diced white onions

1 cup brown rice

2 tbsp. tomato sauce

2 cups chicken stock

Recipe courtesy: Sunfare

PREPARATION:

Put the oil in a medium-size pot and heat briefly over a medium flame. Add the onions and cook for 2 minutes. Add the rice and toss till the rice is coated in oil. Add the tomato sauce and toss again till the rice is red. Add the chicken stock and reduce the heat. Continue simmering till the rice is tender.

Brown Rice Pilaf

INGREDIENTS:

1 tsp. oil

2 tbsp. diced white onions

1 cup brown rice

2 cups chicken stock

2 pieces bay leaf

Recipe courtesy: Sunfare

PREPARATION:

Put the oil in a medium-size pot and heat briefly over a medium flame. Add the onions and cook for 2 minutes. Add the rice and toss till the rice is coated with the oil. Add the chicken stock and the bay leaf. Reduce the heat and simmer for 35–40 minutes or until the rice is tender.

Fried Brown Rice

INGREDIENTS:

1 tsp. minced fresh garlic

1 egg, beaten

2 tbsp. green onion (chopped)

1 cup cooked brown rice

1 tbsp. soy sauce

Recipe courtesy: Sunfare

PREPARATION:

Add the garlic and the egg to a medium-size pot and cook over a medium flame till the egg is set. Add the green onions and the rice; toss till everything is mixed well. Add the soy sauce and toss till the mixture is coated with it.

Roasted New Potatoes

INGREDIENTS:

6 baby red potatoes, cut in half

1 tsp. olive oil

1 tsp. Mrs. Dash

Recipe courtesy: Sunfare

PREPARATION:

Preheat the oven to 350°F. Toss the potatoes in olive oil and Mrs. Dash. Put them in a baking pan and cover with foil. Bake for 40 minutes or until tender; remove the foil and continue baking for 5 minutes. Serve.

Spanish Rice

INGREDIENTS:

1 tsp. oil

¼ cup corn

¼ cup peas

1 cup cooked brown rice

Recipe courtesy: Sunfare

PREPARATION:

Put the oil in a medium-size pot and heat briefly over a medium flame. Add the corn and the peas and cook till coated with oil. Add the rice and toss for 2 more minutes. Serve.

Yam Fries

INGREDIENTS:

1 yam (cut into sticks)

1 tsp. oil

Recipe courtesy: Sunfare

PREPARATION:

Place the yams in the freezer till frozen.

Preheat the oven to 350°F.

Spread the yams on a sprayed cookie sheet and coat in oil. Bake for 40 minutes or until crisp.

Rosemary New Potatoes

INGREDIENTS:

6 baby red potatoes, cut in half

1 tsp. olive oil

1 tsp. Mrs. Dash

1 sprig rosemary, chopped

Recipe courtesy: Sunfare

PREPARATION:

Preheat the oven to 350°F.

Toss the potatoes in the olive oil, Mrs. Dash, and rosemary. Place them in a baking pan and cover with foil. Bake for 40 minutes or until tender; remove the foil and bake for 5 minutes more.

Snacks

Alaskan Seafood Lettuce Cups

Calories: 124

INGREDIENTS:

4 oz. imitation crabmeat

1 tsp. nonfat mayonnaise

½ tsp. wasabi

½ tsp. soy sauce

4 leaves butter leaf lettuce

Recipe courtesy: Sunfare

PREPARATION:

Shred the imitation crab. Add the mayonnaise, wasabi, and soy sauce. Mix together and wrap in lettuce leaves.

SUGARS: 0.73 gram

Caprese Kebab

Calories: 173

INGREDIENTS:

4½ oz. mozzarella balls, part skim

4 cherry tomatoes

4 fresh basil leaves

2 tbsp. pesto

Recipe courtesy: Sunfare

PREPARATION:

Skewer two kebabs in this order:

1. Cherry tomato
2. Basil leaf
3. Mozzarella ball
4. Basil leaf
5. Cherry tomato
6. Basil leaf
7. Mozzarella ball

Drizzle with pesto and serve.

SUGARS: 2.35 grams

Mini Turkey Sliders

Calories: 157

INGREDIENTS:

2 oz. turkey breast (ground)

1 tbsp. barbecue sauce

1 tbsp. Dijon mustard

2 leaves butter leaf lettuce

2 tomatoes, sliced

Recipe courtesy: Sunfare

PREPARATION:

Preheat the oven to 350°F.
Combine the turkey, barbecue
sauce, and Dijon mustard. Form
into two patties and bake 10–15
minutes or until done. Place each
on top of a lettuce leaf and top with
a slice of tomato.

SUGARS: 3.79 grams

Deviled Eggs

Calories: 151

INGREDIENTS:

2 hard-boiled eggs, cut in half and
  hollowed out (reserve yolk)

1 oz. lite Italian dressing

1 tsp. chopped parsley

½ oz. diced turkey bacon

Paprika

Recipe courtesy: Sunfare

PREPARATION:

Cut the eggs in half and gently
scoop out the yolk into a bowl.
Mash the yolk and add enough
salad dressing to get a creamy
consistency. Stir in the parsley and
the chopped-up turkey bacon.
Scoop the filling back into the egg
white. Sprinkle with paprika for
color.

SUGARS: 1.6 grams

Shrimp Cocktail

Calories: 115

INGREDIENTS:

3 small pieces precooked shrimp

1 oz. cocktail sauce

Recipe courtesy: Sunfare

PREPARATION:

Dip the shrimp in the cocktail
sauce and enjoy.

SUGARS: 5.23 grams

Deviled Tomatoes

Calories: 146

INGREDIENTS:

1 tbsp. diced onions

½ hard-boiled egg, diced

1 tbsp. diced celery

1 tsp. relish

1 tbsp. Caesar dressing

Salt and pepper to taste

1 Roma tomato, cut in half and
    hollowed out

Parsley to taste

PREPARATION:

Mix the onions, egg, and celery
with a small amount of relish
and Caesar dressing. Season
with salt and pepper. Scoop into
the hollowed-out Roma pieces.
Garnish with parsley.

SUGARS:

4.07 grams

Recipe courtesy: Sunfare

Grilled BBQ Strips

Calories: 100

INGREDIENTS:

2 oz. chicken breast

Salt and pepper to taste

1 tbsp. barbecue sauce

Recipe courtesy: Sunfare

PREPARATION:

Season the chicken with salt and
pepper. Coat with barbecue sauce,
grill until done, then cut into strips.

SUGARS: 3.1 grams

Grilled Stuffed Zucchini Rolls

Calories: 142

INGREDIENTS:

⅛ zucchini cut into ¼-inch slices

1 tsp. olive oil

Salt and pepper to taste

1 oz. goat cheese

1 tsp. chopped parsley

1 tsp. lemon juice

2 tsp. chopped basil

2 tbsp. chopped fresh spinach leaves

PREPARATION:

Brush the zucchini with olive oil, salt, and pepper. Grill until tender.

Combine the goat cheese, parsley, lemon juice, basil, and spinach. Form this mixture into ½-ounce balls and roll the zucchini around it.

SUGARS: 3.54 grams

Recipe courtesy: Sunfare

Pigs in a Blanket

Calories: 179

INGREDIENTS:

1 oz. yellow mustard

½ 6-inch whole wheat low-carb tortilla

2 oz. turkey dog

Recipe courtesy: Sunfare

PREPARATION:

Preheat the oven to 350°F.

Put mustard on the tortilla. Roll the turkey dog in the tortilla, securing it with a toothpick. Spray lightly with cooking spray.

Bake 10–15 minutes or until the tortilla is light and crispy, and then slice into 2-inch pieces.

SUGARS: 1.75 grams

Pizza Margarita

Calories: 137

INGREDIENTS:

1 6-inch whole wheat tortilla

2 tbsp. marinara sauce

2 oz. part-skim mozzarella cheese

2 tbsp. chopped fresh basil

Italian seasoning to taste

Recipe courtesy: Sunfare

PREPARATION:

Preheat the oven to 350°F.

Coat the tortilla with marinara sauce, then top it with the cheese, basil, and Italian herbs. Bake 10–15 minutes or until the cheese melts and the tortilla is crispy.

SUGARS: 2.28 grams

Sesame Chicken Strips

Calories: 114

INGREDIENTS:

2 oz. chicken breast, cut into strips

1 tsp. sesame seeds

Salt and pepper to taste

2 tbsp. soy sauce

Recipe courtesy: Sunfare

PREPARATION:

Coat the chicken breast in sesame seeds and salt and pepper. Sear until crispy. Serve with a side of soy sauce.

SUGARS: 2 grams

Turkey Skewers

Calories: 91

INGREDIENTS:

2 oz. sliced turkey deli meat,
   cut into 1-inch strips

¼ cup diced red bell pepper

4 cherry tomatoes, halved

1 tsp. lemon pepper

2 tbsp. chipotle mustard

Recipe courtesy: Sunfare

PREPARATION:

Roll up each turkey slice. Place onto skewers in this order: turkey, bell pepper, turkey, cherry tomato. Season the skewers with lemon pepper and grill. Serve with a side of chipotle mustard.

SUGARS: 4.17 grams

Shrimp Seviche

Calories: 86

INGREDIENTS:

2 oz. shrimp

1 oz. diced cucumbers

1 oz. diced tomatotes

1 oz. diced red onions

1 tsp. chopped cilantro

½ lemon

Salt and pepper to taste

PREPARATION:

Cook the shrimp in water. Cool and dice. Mix with the remaining ingredients. Squeeze lemon juice over the mixture, adjust the seasoning, and serve.

SUGARS: 3.45 grams

Recipe courtesy: Sunfare

Turkey Cheese Snack

Calories: 155

INGREDIENTS:

½ 6-inch whole wheat low-carb tortilla

½ tbsp. chipotle mayonnaise

½ oz. turkey, sliced

½ oz. Swiss cheese, sliced

1 tbsp. finely diced celery

1 tbsp. finely diced onions

Recipe courtesy: Sunfare

PREPARATION:

Spread the tortilla with the mayo. Top with the sliced turkey and Swiss cheese. Sprinkle with the diced celery and onions. Roll the tortilla very tightly and slice into ½-inch pieces. One serving is two pieces.

SUGARS: 2.9 grams

Wrap-and-Roll Mini Pinwheels

Calories: 168

INGREDIENTS:

1 6-inch whole wheat low-carb tortilla

½ oz. low-fat cream cheese

1 tsp. chopped parsley

1 tbsp. chopped fresh basil

2 tbsp. canned roasted red pepper

2 oz. (2 slices) turkey

1 tbsp. low-calorie Italian dressing

Recipe courtesy: Sunfare

PREPARATION:

Spread the tortilla with the cream cheese and sprinkle with the chopped parsley. Add a layer of basil leaves to cover the cream cheese. Add a layer of peppers to cover the basil. Top with the turkey deli meat and roll up tightly. Slice into ½-inch sections. One serving is two pieces.

Drizzle with 1 tbsp. low-calorie dressing.

SUGARS: 4.24 grams

Life After the Plan

After you succeed on this plan, going back to anything that resembles an unhealthy life-style is out of the question! Here are some simple strategies to keep you on track—not for the short term, but for the rest of your life.

* Be prepared to eat. Make sure your meals and snacks are pre-prepared and ready to go when it's time to eat; if you wait too long or miss a meal, you can lose energy and disrupt your eating rhythm, which in turn will throw off your body's metabolism. An easy way to do this is to prepare several days' worth of food at once; it's a short time investment up front that will not only save you time and energy down the road, but also set you up for total success!

* Food: Don't leave home without it. Try to always have some type of snack on hand in case you are away from home, stuck in traffic, or just someplace where healthy food is unavailable. If you're going to be traveling by plane, order a special meal so you're not forced to eat something unhealthy. No matter what, do everything you can to avoid fast food or other unhealthy quick fixes.

Appendix B

Using my food guidelines, I've created a meal planner to help you plan and keep track of foods on my 5 + 2 Plan. This planner provides spaces to record what you eat and is organized into one calendar week. Whenever you eat a specific food, simply check off the food in the space provided. This planner can serve as a daily reminder of how well you're doing and make meal planning a breeze. Be sure to draw a smiley face next to meals that were clean and perfect. You won't have to use this tool forever—only until you get the hang of it.

MONDAY   *Date:*

BREAKFAST:

MIDMORNING SNACK:

LUNCH:

MIDAFTERNOON SNACK:

DINNER:

Daily allotments (look over your daily meal plan and check off servings under each nutrient to make sure you've eaten enough of each):

4 PROTEINS   ☐ ☐ ☐ ☐

3 VEGGIES   ☐ ☐ ☐

2 FRUITS   ☐ ☐

2 GRAINS   ☐ ☐

1 FAT   ☐

NOTES:

TUESDAY   *Date:*

BREAKFAST:

MIDMORNING SNACK:

LUNCH:

MIDAFTERNOON SNACK:

DINNER:

Daily allotments (look over your daily meal plan and check off servings under each nutrient to make sure you've eaten enough of each):

4 PROTEINS   ☐ ☐ ☐ ☐

3 VEGGIES   ☐ ☐ ☐

2 FRUITS   ☐ ☐

2 GRAINS   ☐ ☐

1 FAT   ☐

NOTES:

WEDNESDAY   *Date:*

BREAKFAST:

MIDMORNING SNACK:

LUNCH:

MIDAFTERNOON SNACK:

DINNER:

Daily allotments (look over your daily meal plan and check off servings under each nutrient to make sure you've eaten enough of each):

4 PROTEINS   ☐ ☐ ☐ ☐

3 VEGGIES   ☐ ☐ ☐

2 FRUITS   ☐ ☐

2 GRAINS   ☐ ☐

1 FAT   ☐

NOTES:

THURSDAY   *Date:*

BREAKFAST:

MIDMORNING SNACK:

LUNCH:

MIDAFTERNOON SNACK:

DINNER:

Daily allotments (look over your daily meal plan and check off servings under each nutrient to make sure you've eaten enough of each):

4 PROTEINS   ☐ ☐ ☐ ☐

3 VEGGIES   ☐ ☐ ☐

2 FRUITS   ☐ ☐

2 GRAINS   ☐ ☐

1 FAT   ☐

NOTES:

FRIDAY   *Date:*

BREAKFAST:

MIDMORNING SNACK:

LUNCH:

MIDAFTERNOON SNACK:

DINNER:

Daily allotments (look over your daily meal plan and check off servings under each nutrient to make sure you've eaten enough of each):

4 PROTEINS   ☐ ☐☐☐

3 VEGGIES   ☐ ☐☐

2 FRUITS   ☐ ☐

2 GRAINS   ☐ ☐

1 FAT   ☐

NOTES:

SATURDAY   *Date:*

BREAKFAST:

MIDMORNING SNACK:

LUNCH:

MIDAFTERNOON SNACK:

DINNER:

Daily allotments (look over your daily meal plan and check off servings under each nutrient to make sure you've eaten enough of each):

4 PROTEINS   ☐ ☐☐☐

3 VEGGIES   ☐ ☐☐

2 FRUITS   ☐ ☐

2 GRAINS   ☐ ☐

1 FAT   ☐

TREAT MEAL: Please note which meals were treat meals and record the calorie count of each one here:

NOTES:

(SUNDAY)   *Date:*

BREAKFAST:

MIDMORNING SNACK:

LUNCH:

MIDAFTERNOON SNACK:

DINNER:

Daily allotments (look over your daily meal plan and check off servings under each nutrient
to make sure you've eaten enough of each):

4 PROTEINS   ☐ ☐☐☐

3 VEGGIES   ☐ ☐☐

2 FRUITS   ☐ ☐

2 GRAINS   ☐ ☐

1 FAT   ☐

TREAT MEAL: Please note which meals were treat meals and record the calorie count of each one here:

NOTES:

Appendix C

Keeping a regular training log is one of the best ways to make sure you're making progress toward your exercise and fitness goals. This easy-to-use sample log will help you keep track of your daily workouts; your reps, sets, and poundages; your motivation and energy levels; muscle soreness; and overall progress. Writing down your daily exercise in this log makes you mindful of what you're doing and allows you to review your progress after each workout.

Date:

WARM-UP EXERCISES:

EXERCISES	REPS	SETS	POUNDAGES

COOL-DOWN STRETCHES:

CARDIO	MODE	DURATION

NOTES:

Appendix D

Bibliography

CHAPTER 1. IT'S ALL ABOUT CHEMISTRY, BABY

He, K., Zhao, L., et al. 2009. Association of monosodium glutamate intake with overweight in Chinese adults: The INTERMAP Study. *Obesity* 16: 1875–1880.

Lark, S. 2008. *Hormone Revolution*. Mountain View, California: Portola Press.

Rodin, J., Wack, J., Ferrannini, E., and DeFronzo, R.A. 1985. Effect of insulin and glucose on feeding behavior. *Metabolism* 34: 826–831.

Wurtman, R.J., and Wurtman, J. 1995. Brain serotonin, carbohydrate-craving, obesity and depression. *Obesity Research* 4: 477S–480S.

CHAPTER 2. YOU *ARE* A SUGAR ADDICT

Cho, E., Spiegelman, D., Hunter, D.J., Chen, W.Y., Colditz, G.A., Willett, W.C. 2003. Premenopausal dietary carbohydrate, glycemic index, glycemic load, and fiber in relation to risk of breast cancer. *Cancer Epidemiology Biomarkers & Prevention* 12: 1153–1158.

Convit, A., Wolf, O.T., Tarshish, C., and de Leon, M.J. 2003. Reduced glucose tolerance is associated with poor memory performance and hippocampal atrophy among normal elderly. *Proceedings of the National Academy of Sciences of the United States of America* 100: 2019–2022.

Giovannucci, E. 2001. Insulin, insulin-like growth factors and colon cancer: A review of the evidence. *Journal of Nutrition* 131(11 Suppl): 3109S–3120S.

Schwartz, M.B., Vartanian, L.R., Wharton, C.M., and Brownell, K.D. 2008. Examining the nutritional quality of breakfast cereals marketed to children. *Journal of the American Dietetic Association* 108: 702–705.

Tavani, A., Giordano, L., Gallus, S., Talamini, R., Franceschi, S., Giacosa, A., Montella, M., and La Vecchia, C. 2006. Consumption of sweet foods and breast cancer risk in Italy. *Annals of Oncology* 17: 34134–34135.

CHAPTER 3. THREE ORGANS THAT MAKE YOU FAT OR SKINNY

Andrews, K., Schweitzer, A., Zhao, C., et al. 2007. The caffeine contents of dietary supplements commonly purchased in the US: Analysis of 53 products with caffeine-containing ingredients. *Analytical and Bioanalytical Chemistry* 389: 231–239.

Chou, K.H. and Bell, L.N. 2007. Caffeine content of prepackaged national-brand and private-label carbonated beverages. *Journal of Food Science* 72: C337–C342.

CHAPTER 4. ADD TO LOSE: MY 2-WEEK JUMP START

de Oliveira, M.C., Sichieri, R., Venturim, Mozzer, R. 2008. A low-energy-dense diet adding fruit reduces weight and energy intake in women. *Appetite* 51: 291–295.

Johnston, C.S., Beezhold, B.L., Mostow, B., and Swan, P.D. 2007. Plasma vitamin C is inversely related to body mass index and waist circumference but not to plasma adiponectin in nonsmoking adults. *Journal of Nutrition* 137: 1757–1762.

Vander Wal, J.S., Marth, J.M., Khosla, P., Jen, K.L., and Dhurandhar, N.V. 2005. Short-term effect of eggs on satiety in overweight and obese subjects. *Journal of the American College of Nutrition* 24: 510–515.

CHAPTER 5. DEPRIVATION DOESN'T WORK: MY 5 + 2 FOOD PLAN

Hollis, J.F., Gullion, C.M., Stevens, V.J., Brantley, P.J., Appel, L.J., et al. 2008. Weight loss during the intensive intervention phase of the weight-loss maintenance trial. *American Journal of Preventive Medicine* 35: 118–126.

Weigle, D.S., Breen, P.A., Matthys, C.C., Callahan, H.S., Meeuws, K.E., Burden, V.R., and Purnell, J.Q. 2005. A high-protein diet induces sustained reductions in appetite, ad libitum caloric intake, and body weight despite compensatory changes in diurnal plasma leptin and ghrelin concentrations. *American Journal of Clinical Nutrition* 82: 41–48.

CHAPTER 6. GET THIN IN THE REAL WORLD

Fowler, S.P., Williams, K., Resendez, R.G., Hunt, K.J., Hazuda, H.P., and Stern, M.P. 2008. Fueling the obesity epidemic? Artificially sweetened beverage use and long-term weight gain. *Obesity* 16: 1894–1900.

Wansink, B., van Ittersum, K., and Painter, J.E. 2006. Ice cream illusions: Bowls, spoons, and self-served portion sizes. *American Journal of Preventive Medicine* 31: 240–243.

CHAPTER 7. 20 MINUTES TO A FASTER METABOLISM: MY 2-WEEK CARDIO PLAN

Trapp, E.G., Chisholm, D.J., Freund, J., and Boutcher, S.H. 2008. The effects of high-intensity intermittent exercise training on fat loss and fasting insulin levels of young women. *International Journal of Obesity* 32: 684–691.

CHAPTER 8. BUILDING THE PERFECT MACHINE

Schuenke, M.D., Mikat, R.P., and McBride, J.M. 2002. Effect of an acute period of resistance exercise on excess post-exercise oxygen consumption: Implications for body mass management. *European Journal of Applied Physiology* 86: 411–417.

CHAPTER 9. MY FAT-BURNING EXERCISES

Editor. June 2008. Get focused. *Muscle & Fitness.* Accessed online April 2009.

CHAPTER 10. FORM, FUNCTION, FATIGUE: POWER CIRCUITS

Cousins, S.O. 2003. A self-referent thinking model: How older adults may talk themselves out of being physically active. *Health Promotion Practice* 4: 439–448.

CHAPTER 11. METAPHYSIQUES

Crum, A.J., and Langer, E.J. 2007. Mind-set matters: Exercise and the placebo effect. *Psychological Science* 18:165–171.

Richardson, M.A., Post-White, J., Grimm, E.A., Moye, L.A., Singletary, S.E., and Justice, B. 1997. Coping, life attitudes, and immune responses to imagery and group support after breast cancer treatment. *Alternative Therapies in Health and Medicine* 3: 62–70.

Appendix E

WEBSITE: WWW.JACKIEWARNER.COM

If you want to get even more out of my program, I invite you to visit my website at www .jackiewarner.com. Here you can get an up-close and personal look at my world and perhaps learn some new things about diet, exercise, or me. There's a lot to see, so feel free to look around. If you like what you see, you can even join my "Jackie's Club" for additional information on diet, training, and other fitness advice.

JACKIE WARNER DVDs

To enhance your training, check out my DVDs, available through my website:

DVD "Workout" One-On-One Training with Jackie. This DVD features my 20-minute upper body, lower body, and core workouts, which deliver ultimate fat burn and body tone by using my exclusive moves in fusion cardio and strength training.

DVD Personal Training with Jackie: Power Circuit Training. My signature circuit workouts include Power Burn, for ultimate weight loss and accelerated results! There are also five powerful workout options: 15-Minute Total Body Circuit, 40-Minute Total Body

Circuit, 15-Minute Abs Only Circuit, 15-Minute Upper Body Circuit, and 15-Minute Lower Body Circuit. Also included is my 5-Day Noncookers Meal Plan for faster results.

JACKIE WARNER PRODUCTS

10 Clothing. Check out my new clothing line, 10 Clothing, which includes hats, T-shirts, workout pants, and more at www.jackiewarner.com.

WEBSITE: WWW.SUNFARE.COM

All of the recipes in this book were provided by Sunfare, a great way to get daily home delivery of personalized, freshly made meals and family-style dinners. For more information on the many programs they offer, check out their website.

Index

with lemon, 26, 48, 60, 79
quick tip, 61
weight loss. *See also* eating
    plan; metaphysiques
adding foods for, 4, 57–62
eating plan, 67–90
fat-loss goals, 199–201
food deprivation and
    failed, 4, 5, 58, 67–68
hormones that make you
    thin, 14–18
interval intensity training,
    114
metaphysiques, 195–207
positive thinking and,
    199

Power Circuits, 165–92
protein and quicker, 73
resistance training for fast,
    124–25
supplements for, 62–65
three organs that affect,
    40–48
three simple rules, 4
2-week cardio plan, 113–
    22
variety of foods and, 90
vitamin C for, 64
whey protein, 49
BCAAs in, 72
Citrus Power Cleanse
    Protein Shake, 248

8-ounce shake daily, 61
5 + 2 plan, use during, 72
Green Energy Shake, 248
ingredients for shakes, 84
Slim Berry Delight Protein
    Shake, 249
whole grains, 15, 23, 24
selections for daily, 76
shopping for, 99
Wurtman, Judith J., 20

zinc, 15, 25, 51, 62–63
food sources, 15, 25, 69,
    70, 99
zucchini, 59
Grilled Stuffed Rolls, 279

About the Author

Celebrity fitness pioneer Jackie Warner is proof that women can have it all. The successful entrepreneur and television personality has transformed the fitness world and garnered lots of fans along the way.

A Midwestern girl turned self-made millionaire at the age of 22, Jackie was inspired to pursue a career in fitness and nutrition after training a few close friends to dramatic life-changing results. Within a year, Jackie opened her first health center, Lift. The revolutionary fitness facility was the first health club in Southern California to accept health insurance for exercise.

In 2004, Jackie founded Beverly Hills–based Sky Sport & Spa. Employing Jackie's complete approach to fitness, Sky Sport is the nation's premiere full-service wellness practice. Although frequented by fitness aficionados for years, Sky Sport was introduced to the rest of the world on Jackie's hit television show, *Work Out*.

A docudrama about Jackie's work and private life, *Work Out*, chronicled Jackie's personal triumphs and challenges while running a multimedia fitness empire and navigating the often topsy-turvy world of romance. Fans were hooked. Jackie's loving-yet-tough demeanor resonated with audiences across the world. She is now the star and executive producer of her sophomore Bravo series, *Thintervention*.

Jackie is the co-founder of the country's premiere and only intensive luxury fitness vacation, SkyLab. Personally overseen by Jackie, SkyLab is a six-night, seven-day life-changing fitness retreat. Participants attend fitness-education seminars, receive specialized nutritional counseling, and undergo group therapy that emphasizes critical areas, like overcoming personal challenges and goal setting.

Jackie can also add the titles of DVD star and author to her résumé. She currently stars in the bestselling DVD *ONE-ON-ONE Training with Jackie* and just released her highly anticipated second DVD, *Personal Training with Jackie: Power Circuit Training.*

Jackie will also soon be launching her next business endeavor, Jackie Warner Fitness.